Coping with Caesarean and Other Difficult Births

Fran Reader
and
Wendy Savage

WITH A FOREWORD BY
CLAIRE RAYNER

Macdonald Publishers, Edinburgh

ISBN 0 86334 019 9 (Hardback)
ISBN 0 86334 001 6 (Paperback)

Published by
Macdonald Publishers, Edinburgh
Edgefield Road, Loanhead,
Midlothian EH20 9SY

Design and cover by Iain McKinlay
Illustrations by Sue Innes

Printed in Scotland by
Macdonald Printers (Edinburgh) Limited
Edgefield Road, Loanhead,. Midlothian

Coping with Caesarean
and Other Difficult Births

Contents

For Christine and Kate

Foreword

No matter how many important things a woman does in her life—be it climbing the Matterhorn, writing a symphony or making a home—she will never feel more involved in the act of creation than when she is having a baby. And unless she is a very unusual or very unhappy woman she'll want to make as good a job as she can of her motherhood. Women are, by and large, enormously self-sacrificing during pregnancy and labour; they take excellent care of their babies long before they are born. The reward they most hope for is a healthy baby—and for themselves an exciting, not too arduous birth-giving experience.

And for the vast majority, that is precisely what they have. But there are some who do not, and this book is written for them. It's a superb book, solid with information and honestly presented. It tells it as it is, without glossing over the unpleasantness of the difficult birth, yet manages to do so without being unduly alarming. And that is no mean feat.

Like every midwife I wish every mother a peaceful, joyous pregnancy, and a normal, spontaneous delivery of her healthy baby—but just in case delivery turns out for you to be a rather more complex business than you anticipated, read this book. You can lose nothing by gaining knowledge, and you may be very grateful indeed, if you turn out to be one of the five to ten per cent of mothers who need a Caesarean section, or the five to ten per cent who need a forceps delivery, that you did so. Your reading will help you cope with it all—and therefore to have that healthy baby you're working to hard to create.

Claire Rayner
London, April 1983

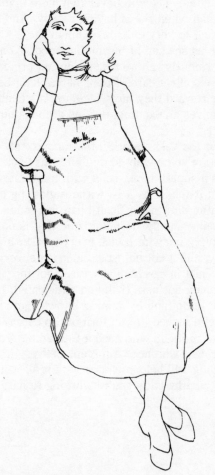

The last few days of waiting
can seem terribly long

Introduction

The birth of a child should be one of life's crowning experiences, the culmination of nine months waiting and the beginning of parenthood. But nature does not always get it right and not all births can be normal deliveries through the mother's vagina (birth passage). Medical assistance with the birth is then necessary to rescue the baby or mother from impending disaster. Between five and ten per cent of babies are born by Caesarean section, which is an operation to deliver the baby through the mother's abdomen: another five to ten per cent of babies will be assisted through the vagina with forceps or a vacuum extractor. Three to four per cent of babies will be breech (bottom) first in the womb; some of these will be born vaginally and some will be Caesarean births. Thus there is a spectrum of ways of giving birth, with or without assistance, and each way can be a success story all of its own.

We hope this book will help dispel some of the fear of the unknown, and give you positive support to help cope, and participate fully, if you should find that the birth of one of your babies is a difficult one.

Every hospital will have different ways of dealing with difficult births and within the hospital it is probable that the ideas and practices of individual doctors will differ. In this book we have tried to combine the ideas and techniques that we have seen or practised ourselves. We would advise you to ask your midwife and doctor what to expect in your own hospital.

The authors are grateful for the help of Gill Mathews, who did most of the typing, and Mary Alexander, Carol Avery, Ruth-Mary Burch, Patricia Egan, Carol Febry, Helen Keeley, Sue Peters, Lenda Poole, Jackie Sanderson, Janet Tarbun and Lynn Woods, who all contributed either as patients or as friends.

Frances Reader
Wendy Savage
February, 1983

Coping with Caesarean

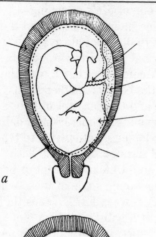

a

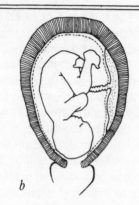

b

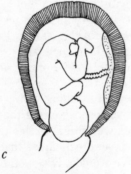

c

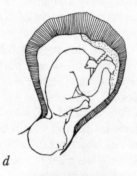

d

The stages of labour:

a) *The contractions start (1st stage)*
b) *The cervix begins to dilate*
c) *The head starts to come through the cervix (2nd stage)*
d) *The head is coming through the vagina*
e) *The afterbirth comes away (3rd stage)*

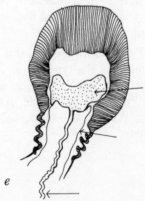

e

1 Normal Labour and Pain Relief in Labour

Most hospitals run their own antenatal classes and give you the opportunity to look around the maternity unit; this can be an ideal time to ask the questions you forgot to ask in the fraught environment of a busy antenatal clinic.

Don't forget that your GP may be the best person to approach with your questions. Sometimes the GP can liaise with the hospital doctor on your behalf.

The way that a hospital operates and doctors manage childbirth is always changing; but it is possible to lose touch with the changing expectations of the community, or for the community to misunderstand medical practice. We need much better communication between the medical profession and the consumer. If you feel really strongly about problems you have encountered in the system, then please criticise constructively if possible; or you may wish to praise and thank the staff rather than complain. In either case, you could write to the individual concerned, your consultant, the midwifery superintendent, hospital administrators, or local Community Health Council.

Before looking at what can go wrong, let us look at what happens in normal labour and consider the choices of pain relief available.

Labour is the process whereby the uterus (womb) contracts regularly to open the cervix (neck of the womb) and push the baby through the birth canal. The active first stage of labour is reckoned from the onset of regular painful contractions which also open up the cervix; this may be preceded by a latent period where the contractions are thinning the cervix but not opening it. The second stage of labour starts when the cervix is fully open and the baby passes through the birth canal to be born. The third stage of labour is the delivery of the placenta (afterbirth) and membranes.

It can be difficult to be certain when labour actually begins. Sometimes the waters break before painful contractions start and sometimes after. Sometimes the blood-stained mucus plug from the cervix (the 'show') comes away several days before labour begins and sometimes the show and the painful contractions come together. You should always go to hospital or call your midwife if you think the waters have broken, and painful contractions coming on average at least every ten minutes for one hour usually mean you are in labour; sometimes contractions start by coming every 2-4 minutes, in which case you will not be in doubt!

Contractions are almost always very painful, even in a normal birth, though some women experience little pain. On average, contractions in the early part of the first stage of

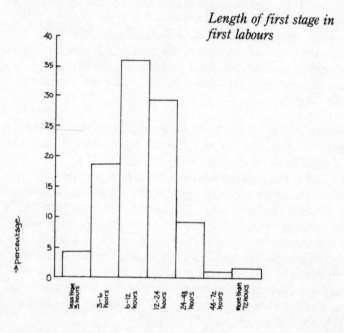

Length of first stage in first labours

labour last about 30 seconds and come every 5-10 minutes. They build up to last 50-60 seconds and come every 2-3 minutes late in the first stage. Sometimes, just before the cervix is fully open, you get a strong desire to push with each contraction, as if opening your bowels; in other labours the desire to push does not start until you are well into the second stage. First labours differ from subsequent labours in that the first stage and second stage are longer, as the table shows. Thus there is a spectrum of what happens in normal labour and there is a choice of pain relief to help different women cope with their individual experiences.

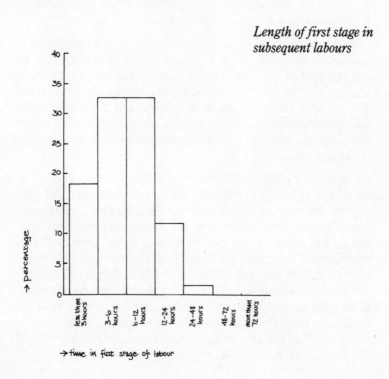

Length of first stage in subsequent labours

Pain Relief

Preparing your body with sleep and nutritious food will help you to cope with labour. The pain you feel during labour can be heightened by fear, so if possible attend antenatal relaxation classes at your hospital, National Childbirth Trust (NCT) classes, yoga or something similar. You will learn a lot about your body, how to relax, how to breathe through the contractions and what is likely to happen to you. This knowledge will help give you confidence and dispel the fear.

Some women find that, with the support of their partner and/or midwife, their relaxation and breathing techniques are sufficient for them to cope with the pain. If you need extra assistance there are three possibilities—

Gas and Oxygen (Entonox). This is a mixture you breathe, and you can control how much you take. It can be very helpful for the last part of the first stage of labour. It is best to start using the Entonox at the very beginning of a contraction, because it will not take effect for about 20 seconds and this should then coincide with the strongest part of the contraction. The gas is nitrous oxide and although it is sometimes called 'laughing gas' it can also make you cry!

Opiates, e.g. Pethidine. This is an injection given into the muscle of your thigh or bottom which will make you feel drowsy and help you relax between contractions. It tends to enhance your mood, so it helps if you feel positive about having Pethidine, rather than depressed about 'giving in'. It is useful if you need pain relief early in the first stage. If given close to delivery time it can make the baby drowsy, but this can be dealt with by giving the baby an injection to counteract this effect. In some hospitals, Diamorphine is used instead of Pethidine. Both Pethidine and Diamorphine can cause vomiting. It is not unccommon to be sick in labour anyway. If this occurs, an antisickness injection can be given.

Normal Labour

Epidural Anaesthetic An epidural is a type of local anaesthetic used to block sensation in certain nerves. It is similar to the local anaesthetic used by dentists to numb a tooth before putting in a filling. The nerves being blocked by the epidural are those carrying the sensation of labour pains from the uterus to the spinal cord and thus to the brain. It is impossible to block the nerves sensing pain without also blocking some of the nerves carrying messages to the muscles of the legs. It is therefore common for a woman to feel weakness from the waist down if she has an epidural. Blood vessels in the legs also open up, which can cause a drop in blood pressure and can make the legs feel warm.

An epidural anaesthetic is set up by an anaesthetist or sometimes an obstetrician with anaesthetic training. It takes at least 10 minutes to get the epidural set up, and another 10-20 minutes for it to become effective and relieve pain. An epidural can be very helpful if you feel you have a low pain threshold or if it is suspected that you may have a long labour (see Page 29). It can be used for delivery with forceps or ventouse (see Pages 53-7) and for a Caesarean birth, but not where a time delay could be critical (see Page 48).

A doctor will put up a drip first and give you extra fluids through your vein. This helps your body to cope with the drop in blood pressure (see above). Your pulse and blood pressure are checked at the beginning. You will then be helped to lie on your side on the edge of a firm bed and to curl into a ball. Some anaesthetists prefer you sitting upright on the bed with your back towards them and your legs hanging over the other side of the bed. Either position helps to display the knobbles of your spine but can be difficult to hold during contractions. Your partner can help you but he may be asked to wait outside while the epidural is set up; if so, enlist a nurse or midwife to help you relax and stay in position—this makes it easier for the anaesthetist. Everyone differs in their ability to perform a task while being watched; some doctors feel at ease but some

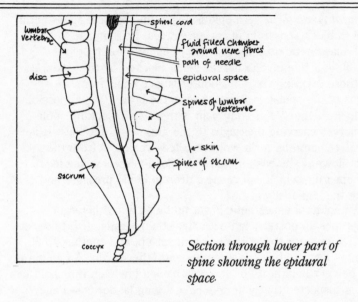

lumbar vertebrae

spinal cord

disc

fluid filled chamber around nerve fibres

path of needle

epidural space

spines of lumbar vertebrae

skin

spines of sacrum

sacrum

coccyx

Section through lower part of spine showing the epidural space.

perform less well, therefore if your partner is asked to leave at any stage this may be disappointing but it will be temporarily necessary. Once you are in position, the anaesthetist washes his hands thoroughly and puts on sterile gloves; he/she then cleans your back with an antispetic and injects some local anaesthetic into your back, to numb the spot where the epidural will go.

Once the local anaesthetic is working, he/she then pushes another needle into your back, advancing it slowly until the epidural space is reached. This is a space inside your bony spinal column but before the spinal cord itself. The epidural space is crossed by the nerves as they leave the spinal cord to pass out between each of the vertebrae (see diagram). When the needle is being advanced you will be aware of the pushing, and perhaps some discomfort. Occasionally a sharp pain will be felt; if so, you must tell the doctor as this information is important to help place the epidural correctly.

Normal Labour

Once the needle is in place, a thin plastic tube is threaded through it into the epidural space, and the needle itself removed. The plastic tube (epidural catheter) is about three feet long but only about three inches are left inside your back; the rest of the tube remains outside and is brought up your back and over one shoulder. It is stuck in place with waterproof Elastoplast or similar tape. The end of your catheter has a small filter attached to it, into which a syringe will fit to inject more local anaesthetic.

Once the epidural is in place, you can straighten up to lie more comfortably on your side and your pulse, blood pressure and baby's heart-beat will be checked.

The anaesthetist may well begin by injecting a small amount of local anaesthetic called a test dose. Very occasionally there may be an excessive drop in your blood pressure, and this will be picked up by the test dose. No harm is done, because the drip can correct this, but the full dose cannot be given. An alternative form of pain relief or anaesthetic will be arranged instead. If all is well after the test dose, the full dose is given, and gradually over the next 10-20 minutes the pain of the contractions disappears and usually your legs become heavy, numb and warm. You may also experience a tingling sensation and develop the shakes—this is similar to shivering after a swim, but doesn't last long.

A nurse will be checking your pulse and blood pressure from time to time and checking the baby's heartbeat. You may be turned to lie for a few minutes on your left side, then a few minutes on your right side to distribute the anaesthetic effect evenly. If the epidural is needed for a Caesarean birth you may be tilted slightly head down, and if it is needed for a forceps delivery you may be sat upright for a while: this helps the local anaesthetic to bathe the nerves to your uterus and abdomen which come from higher up the spinal cord or the nerves to your vagina and bottom which come from lower down.

Occasionally it fails completely, and sometimes the effect is partial. All doctors who do obstetric epidurals are experienced, but some will obviously be more experienced than others, and even very experienced doctors can have failures or partial failures; this is because the anatomy of the backbone varies in each individual and minute variations in the shape of the spine or position of the nerves can mean that the local anaesthetic cannot reach all the right nerves. If this happens, a second try with the epidural will usually overcome the problem if you are prepared to undergo the whole procedure again—it could well be worth it!

During labour, the aneasthetic effect of the epidural lasts for anything from one to four hours. When the effects begin to wear off, more local anaesthetic is injected through the epidural catheter, and you will again be helped to move from side to side and your pulse, blood pressure and baby's heartbeat recorded from time to time.

It is difficult to pass urine with an epidural because you are unaware that you want to. It is important to keep the bladder empty, to give the baby's head room to fit into your pelvis. The reflex reaction to a full bladder may also cause a damping down of contractions. It may be necessary to have a catheter passed to empty your bladder.

This may all seem as though epidurals are fairly plain sailing; as with anything else, however, there can be problems. If you are grossly overweight, if your back is swollen with retained fluid, or if for some reason you cannot curl up sufficiently, then it may prove impossible to set up the epidural.

Certain medical points must also be considered before you have an epidural. If you are taking anticoagulants to thin your blood (usually because of a clot in a vein or a replacement heart valve) then it is usually considered unsafe to perform an epidural. If you have a condition of the nerves, such as multiple sclerosis, or of your backbone, there may be considerable discussion before the decision is taken.

Normal Labour

As we have said, the epidural can sometimes cause a fall in blood pressure. This can be very useful if the doctors are worried by high blood pressure in the mother, but sometimes the fall can affect the flow of blood to the placenta and hence to the baby. As explained previously, the drip can be used to help counteract this problem, but for a short time you may need to breathe oxygen from a mask to help your baby while the blood pressure picks up.

Sometimes the needle goes beyond the epidural space into the space where the spinal column is bathed in fluid. If this happens a dural tap is said to have occurred and the needle needs replacing into the epidural space. Pain relief is still usually effective but if the fluid leaks out from around the spinal cord into the epidural space, this can cause a headache. After delivery you will have to lie flat for 24-48 hours and you will be encouraged to take extra fluids to help to prevent this headache by replacing the fluid. In some countries anaesthetists prefer to enter this fluid-filled space routinely. This is called a spinal anaesthetic; it gives the same pain relief as an epidural, but there can be a greater drop in blood pressure at the time and also top-ups cannot be given, so this procedure is less helpful for long labours.

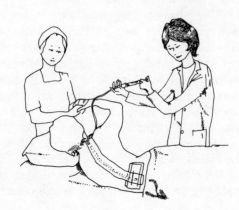

*Topping up
the epidural*

Coping with Caesarean

An epidural may take away sensation during the second stage of labour, which may make it difficult to push effectively with your contractions, and you may miss the sensation of the baby's head and body actually leaving your body. Providing you and the baby are in good condition it is possible to let the effects of the epidural wear off as you enter the second stage of labour and then you do not miss out on these sensations. If you feel you cannot cope with this, or if there is a problem with the baby getting tired in the second stage, then the epidural can be topped up and the birth assisted with forceps or ventouse (see Pages 53-7).

After an epidural anaesthetic there have been cases of continuous back-ache over the site of the epidural; this is usually temporary but can last for up to three months. It may need to be checked by a back specialist if it lasts this long. Occasionally there may be a temporary weakness in one leg. It is difficult to know if the epidural is responsible, because similar temporary weaknesses are seen after labour without an epidural, caused by the baby pressing against a nerve to the leg for a long time, or sometimes forceps may bruise the nerve. These weaknesses are always temporary. They may last up to three months, but with the help of physiotherapy, and in time, full power will always be regained.

There have occasionally been cases of permanent paralysis where human error in management of the epidural is invariably responsible. Such disasters are fortunately rare and in terms of permanent paralysis it is statistically much safer to have an epidural anaesthetic than to cross the road. In the light of past tragedies numerous precautions are taken to avoid such an accident. However, an epidural is never the only way out. If you are truly afraid of the possible complications, then you do not have to have an epidural. Your labour and delivery will still be managed by the doctors and midwives to the best of their ability. Relief of your pain, reassurance of your fears, and a safe outcome for you both can still be achieved.

Normal Labour

Not all hospitals have sufficient numbers of anaesthetists trained in obstetric epidurals to provide an epidural service 24 hours a day. If you are thinking of requesting an epidural then this should be discussed in advance with your consultant.

2 Why Me?

It is normal to expect the whole birth experience to be natural, straightforward, and fulfilling. Unfortunately nature is not always perfect; what are the difficulties and why do doctors need to intervene from time to time? Medical intervention may be necessary before labour begins. It may be safer to encourage labour to start (induction of labour) before any anticipated problems occur. Sometimes it is better if labour does not occur at all, in which case a Caesarean birth can be planned in advance. A Caesarean birth planned in advance is referred to as an Elective Caesarean, whereas a Caesarean performed urgently either before or during labour is referred to as an Emergency Caesarean. If it is safer for the baby or mother to have a short second stage of labour then forceps or ventouse can be used or an episiotomy alone may be necessary if it is safer to speed things up.

Induction of Labour

The place of induction of labour is still contentious. In the mid-1970s it was performed frequently, usually to avoid pregnancy going past 40 weeks or 'term'. Term is the average length of a pregnancy and is about 40 weeks (280 days) from the first day of the mother's last period. This will give you the expected date of delivery but for this date to be reliable, the first day of the last period must be certain and the woman's periods before that time must have been regular every four weeks; so you can see why it is not uncommon for this date to be uncertain. Sometimes the induction did not work and Caesarean sections were performed unnecessarily, which made both the professionals and the consumer groups question such medical intervention.

Induction still has a part to play but each woman and her baby need individual consideration and the risks of the pregnancy continuing need to be weighed up against the risks of induction. Usually the main consideration is how well the placenta is feeding the baby and transferring oxygen. The baby in the uterus is known medically as the fetus; it needs oxygen to survive. If the oxygen supply is poor then the baby will not grow well. Eventually its blood becomes too acid and the heartrate will show changes which suggest that the baby is in danger—'fetal distress'.

The placenta may begin to function less efficiently if the pregnancy lasts more than 294 days and therefore the well-being of the baby must be checked if the pregnancy is to continue, but many doctors prefer to induce labour at this stage. In some women over 35, and certainly over 40, the placenta may begin to fail earlier, at about 280 days.

If a previous baby was stillborn, or died soon after birth, because of lack of oxygen then the next labour may be induced earlier or the baby delivered by Elective Caesarean to try to avoid the same tragedy.

The mother's health may affect the placenta, especially high blood pressure or diabetes. High blood pressure in pregnancy is probably the most common reason for a pregnant woman being admitted to hospital and is also a common reason for inducing labour. High blood pressure can exist before pregnancy but more frequently it is associated with pregnancy and gets better after the birth. This is called pre-eclamptic toxaemia (PET) and may be accompanied by excessive weight gain (more than 26 lbs (12 kg) over the pregnancy), swelling of the ankles and fingers (oedema) and protein in the urine.

If the blood pressure goes too high it can affect the placenta and slow down the baby's growth or cause the placenta to separate from the uterus, causing sudden pain in the abdomen and bleeding from the vagina. It can also harm the mother, causing fits (eclampsia). The baby may be small and not growing well; this may be suspected if the mother has not put on much weight. Women who smoke tend to have smaller babies and if the baby itself is not quite normal it may grow poorly.

The doctor can check the baby's wellbeing during pregnancy. If poor growth is suspected then this can be checked with an ultrasound scan; this is a method of measuring the size of the baby and checking for some major abnormalities by using high frequency sound waves which we cannot hear; the picture of the baby is produced by recording the echoes. The doctor can also check a hormone in the mother's urine or blood called oestriol; falling levels suggest a failing placenta.

The mother herself may suspect the problem if the baby becomes less active. All babies have periods of activity and rest, but several days of reduced or no activity may be important. Finally the baby's heart rate can be checked with a monitor machine (CTG—cardiotocograph) to detect abnormal patterns, which suggest that the baby is distressed.

Monitoring during Labour

If the doctor or midwife suspects that the placenta has not been working well towards the end of pregnancy or if the liquor (water) is stained with meconium (indicating that the

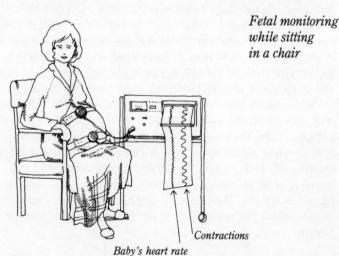

Fetal monitoring while sitting in a chair

Contractions

Baby's heart rate

baby has had its bowels open, which may be a sign of distress) then it will be necessary to watch the effect of the contractions on the baby's heart rate throughout labour. During each contraction the amount of oxygen reaching the baby is reduced, so as labour progresses the baby may become distressed. Some doctors favour monitoring all labours unless the mother expressly requests otherwise; this is because occasionally the most straightforward pregnancy and labour can lead to fetal distress if, for example, the cord is around the baby's neck.

Unfortunately, monitoring the baby's heart beat is associated with lying in bed attached to wires and machines. If this is necessary you can help yourself by keeping as upright as possible, either propped up in bed or sitting out in a chair. If you want to be flatter it is important to lie on one side or the other as this will keep the weight of the uterus off the main vessels in your body carrying oxygen to the placenta, and it also helps improve the quality of the contractions in a similar way to being upright. Some hospitals have telemetry, which is a radio wave system which allows the baby's heart rate to be monitored while you are walking about. It is hoped that this will eventually be available in all obstetric units.

Intervention before Labour

When vaginal delivery is impossible or unsafe for mother or baby an Elective Caesarean birth will be planned.

Not enough room for the baby (cephalo-pelvic disproportion)

If it is obvious that the baby will not come through the mother's pelvis then it will be born by Elective Caesarean. This may be due to the size or position of the baby or the size or shape of the mother's pelvis. Women under five feet tall tend to have a smaller pelvis; in other cases the pelvis may have an abnormal shape, if for example the mother has previously had a fractured pelvis, or had polio when she was a child.

Fibroids or an Ovarian Cyst in the way

These may block the birth passage, so an Elective Caesarean birth is necessary. An ovarian cyst can be removed at the same time but fibroids are best left alone as they will shrink, and if necessary can be removed later when they are smaller.

Problems with the baby

If the baby is in danger of dying during labour because the placenta is not working well then an Elective Caesarean will be performed; sometimes the decision is taken as a matter of urgency.

If there have been problems with a previous stillborn baby or if there have been many years of infertility then it may be considered safer to deliver the baby by an Elective Caesarean, especially if there are any doubts about a vaginal birth.

Problems with the mother's health

Very high blood pressure (see Page 23) can develop after 24 weeks of pregnancy, especially between 28 and 34 weeks, and it may be better for the mother and baby to deliver the baby by Caesarean.

If the mother has previously suffered a stroke, a rise in blood pressure with pushing could be dangerous; occasionally other medical problems such as diabetes or heart disease may have given problems during the pregnancy such that the doctors will advise a Caesarean birth.

Problems with the placenta

(a) A placenta lying across the cervix is called *placenta praevia* and will block the passage of the baby and cause heavy bleeding. Usually the first sign of placenta praevia is bleeding from the vagina which can occur without any pain in the abdomen. The position of the placenta is confirmed by ultrasound and then an Elective Caesarean will be necessary when the baby is mature, at about 38 weeks, or earlier as an emergency if the bleeding is too heavy.

(b) Part of the placenta may peel away from the uterus, causing sudden pain in the abdomen and bleeding from the vagina. This is called a *placental abruption* and is more likely to occur in a mother with high blood pressure. If there is only a small amount of bleeding, it often settles and the pregnancy will be allowed to continue and tests will be done to see if the placenta is still transferring enough oxygen to the baby. If the bleeding is heavy the baby may need rescuing urgently by an Emergency Caesarean. Sometimes the baby dies in which case the doctors will try to induce labour and deliver the dead baby through the vagina.

It is important to report to a doctor straight away if you have any bleeding from the vagina in pregnancy.

Previous surgery to the uterus, cervix or vagina

A previous classical Caesarean scar is weak (see Page 40) and an Elective Caesarean will be necessary next time.

Sometimes a woman may have had an operation to remove part of the cervix to investigate possible pre-cancer. This operation is called a *cone biopsy* and it can leave the cervix weak so that it may open too early and the baby be born prematurely. If this is the case then the cervix can be strengthened with a stitch which is put in under general anaesthetic at about 16 weeks and removed at 38 weeks of pregnancy. Sometimes, however, the cervix becomes very scarred and cannot open during labour.

Following a previous difficult birth through the vagina, the uterus and vagina may have dropped downwards (*prolapse*) and an operation to rectify this may have been done, in which case it is better to deliver any subsequent babies by Elective Caesarean.

Herpes Infections of the Vagina

Herpes is an infection caused by a virus which is similar to the cold sore virus. Similar ulcers can occur around the labia, inside the vagina and on the cervix. These are painful the first time they appear but they may come and go and be less painful after the first attack.

If you have had a herpes infection of the vagina you must tell your obstetrician so that your cervix and vagina can be checked at about 36 weeks of pregnancy. If you have no ulcers it will be safe for your baby to pass through the vagina but if ulcers are present it will be safer for the baby to be born by Elective Caesarean; otherwise it can be infected by the ulcers, and a herpes infection in a new-born baby can be serious.

Intervention during Labour

The baby needs help (fetal distress)

Understanding the importance of the placenta transferring oxygen to the baby helps to explain why an emergency Caesarean may be performed in labour for what is termed 'fetal distress'. This means that the baby is in danger of dying during labour from lack of oxygen unless it is rescued quickly. If the baby becomes distressed during the second stage of labour, it can be rescued using forceps or ventouse, or sometimes the birth can be speeded up with the help of an episiotomy.

The pattern of the baby's heart-rate in response to the contractions will change as the baby becomes distressed. The baby may also open its bowels and pass meconium in response to stress. This will colour the liquid greeny/brown.

If fetal distress is suspected, the acidity and amount of oxygen in the baby's blood can be measured by sampling a very small quantity of blood directly from the baby.

Why Me?

Another cause of fetal distress is prolapse of the umbilical cord. The cord, which carries blood (and hence oxygen) between the placenta and the baby, may slip past the baby into the birth canal when the waters break. This can cause severe distress and if it happens before the cervix is fully open then the baby will need to be born by Caesarean. While preparations are made for the operation, a midwife or doctor will keep a hand inside the vagina to make sure the baby does not lie on the cord. Sometimes the mother may be asked to kneel and keep her bottom up and head down (kow-tow position). This is uncomfortable, but can be life saving for the baby. If this happens in the second stage of labour, the baby can be delivered speedily with forceps.

The baby gets stuck, or labour is protracted

The idea of a baby being born through your vagina may seem quite alarming. It is not unusual to fear that the vagina and pelvis are too small, but late in pregnancy your body prepares for labour and the pelvic joints become softer so they can stretch slightly and provide more room for the baby to come through. Cases where there really is not enough room are referred to medically as *cephalo-pelvic disproportion* (CPD). This may be due to the size or position of the baby, the size of the mother's bony pelvis, or a combination of both factors.

Sometimes the problem is obvious and a Caesarean can be planned in advance, but more commonly the problem is suspected because the baby's head has not gone into the pelvis (engaged) towards the end of the pregnancy. This is an important sign in a first pregnancy but not so important in subsequent pregnancies.

When the problem is suspected the size of your baby is assessed by the doctor examining your abdomen and then measurements can be taken using ultrasound. The size of your bony pelvis is checked during an internal examination and direct measurements can be taken from an X-ray of your pelvis (pelvimetry). (X-rays should be avoided in early pregnancy when the baby is being formed but in late pregnancy they are safer.) The labour is watched carefully and most babies that are not engaged before labour descend easily and are born normally. If the baby does not descend then labour could go on and on and still the cervix not open fully, so the decision is made to deliver by Caesarean.

The Face-Up Baby. Usually the baby comes with the back of its head (occiput) facing forwards. This is the normal occipito-anterior (OA) position, but it is not uncommon, especially with first babies, for the baby to lie with the back of its head towards the mother's back—the occipito-posterior (OP) position. In this position the contractions encourage the baby's head to fall back rather than bend forwards with its chin on its chest (see Fig.). This in turn means that a wider part of the head comes through which may well get stuck, leading to a long labour where both mother and baby become tired. The contractions are often felt as severe backache, and may be irregular and inefficient. Keeping upright will encourage the baby to descend and turn forwards, but after a long painful labour it can be difficult to keep upright. An epidural can be very helpful under these circumstances. Good pain relief makes it easier for the contractions to be improved using a drip with the hormone Syntocinon (see Page 34).

The baby coming breech (bottom), face, brow or shoulder first. It is normal for the top of the baby's head (vertex) to come through the birth canal first. Any other position is considered abnormal and referred to as an *abnormal presentation.* If the baby is lying sideways or if the brow is coming first then the baby cannot get through and must be born by a Caesarean. When the baby is coming bottom or face first it can sometimes be born normally. A baby born face first will have a very bruised and swollen face, but this will settle over 24-48 hours. (For breech first babies, see Page 61.)

Why Me?

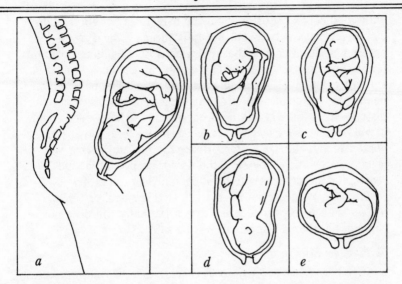

a) A good starting position
b), c) Coming bottom first

d), e) Brow and transverse
presentations will need to be
'rescued' by a Caesarean

Poor Contractions. Long labours with slow progress may be due to weak, irregular contractions; this is more common both in first labours and in women who have had four or more babies. It can also occur when the baby is in the face up position. Such long labours can be very demoralising. A drip containing the hormone Syntocinon will help to improve the contractions, and an epidural may be helpful to see the mother through to a normal or forceps delivery.

A Long Second Stage of Labour. This problem can occur if the contractions become weak or infrequent, in which case a Syntocinon drip will be helpful. Sometimes the mother is too tired to push effectively, or she may be pushing really well with good contractions and still the baby does not come. This can mean that the baby has not fully turned around to the anterior position or else that it is a tight fit. Changing position for pushing may help, especially if you can get upright by squatting, kneeling, or using a birthing stool. The baby will need to be watched carefully to make sure that it does not get distressed. If there is still no progress, or the baby needs help, it will be necessary to have some assistance with forceps or ventouse, and the joint efforts of the mother and doctor will usually succeed. If, however, the doctor suspects that the reason for the delay is a tight fit then he/she can either recommend a Caesarean birth, even at this stage, or try to deliver with forceps, accepting that if the baby still does not come easily then a Caesarean will be safer.

A Previous Scar in the Uterus

If you have had a previous Caesarean or other surgery, such as an operation to remove fibroids, or a hysterotomy (a method of terminating a pregnancy by performing a Caesarean-like operation very early on), then your uterus has a scar in it and such scars may weaken with prolonged labour. Labour is therefore watched very carefully to ensure that progress is normal. Very rarely, the scar may give way, and if the doctor suspects this has happened, then an Emergency Caesarean is performed. The old saying 'Once a Caesarean, always a Caesarean', no longer stands; providing the mother is checked and the pelvis found to be a good shape and size then she may well deliver normally next time (see Page 89).

Note: This is not the case with a previous classical Caesarean scar (see Page 40) which will definitely be too weak.

Problems with the Mother's Health

If the mother's blood pressure has been high during pregnancy, it tends to rise even further with painful contractions and pushing, and this may be dangerous for the mother. The doctor may advise an epidural to help counteract this (see Page 15) and then a forceps or ventouse delivery will help to shorten the second stage. With other medical problems, such as some forms of heart disease, pushing can be harmful to the mother and then forceps are again indicated.

3 What Happens

Induction of Labour

Methods of Induction

Nowadays, most obstetric units have prostaglandin pessaries or jelly which, when placed into the vagina close to the cervix, release the hormone prostaglandin which is the same hormone produced by the uterus at the beginning of natural labour. This hormone is absorbed by the cervix and will frequently trigger off labour. The effectiveness of the prostaglandin depends on whether the uterus is ready to start labour. The state of the cervix will be a good indicator; if it is short, soft and already opening it is said to be favourable or ripe, whereas the reverse is unfavourable or unripe. When the cervix is unfavourable, the prostaglandin pessaries may be used to speed up the process of ripening the cervix ready for labour.

Labour can also be induced by breaking the waters and starting a Syntocinon drip. Breaking the waters is referred to as artificial rupture of membranes (ARM). This is sometimes done with your legs in stirrups in the lithotomy position (so called because it was the original position used for removing bladder stones—Lithos is Greek for stone). Otherwise it can be done with your legs relaxed apart, as for a vaginal examination.

The doctor (or midwife) puts on a protective plastic apron, washes his hands thoroughly and puts on sterile gloves. Then he will clean the area around the entrance to the vagina (the vulva) with a warm antiseptic solution. He will then examine you internally to feel through the cervix for the membranes stretched over the baby's head. This examination can be uncomfortable, but there is no need to worry about it. The membranes themselves do not have sensation so the actual moment of breaking the membranes is not painful. This is done with either a small plastic crochet-like hook or a special metal clip with scissor-like handles. Once the waters have broken you will feel a gush of warm fluid flowing from your vagina. The fluid will be checked to see if it is clear or stained greeny-brown with meconium. Meconium is the substance in the baby's bowels and sometimes the baby will open its bowels before it is born, especially if it is distressed.

Syntocinon Drip

In order to put up a drip the doctor or midwife will need to see the veins on your forearm and back of your hand. He/she may use a tight band or ask an assistant to squeeze your arm; either method will make the veins stand out. Sometimes a small amount of local anaesthetic is injected over the site where the drip will be inserted. The needle which goes into the vein is similar to the needle used when taking blood, except that it has a plastic outer covering. Once inside the vein the pressure on your arm is released and the doctor removes the metal part of the needle leaving the soft plastic part inside the vein with a wider end outside. The drip is then connected to the part outside and the whole thing secured with tape.

The drip is normally placed in such a way that you can still move your fingers and wrist: if this is not possible then your hand and forearm will be gently bandaged to a small board, thus preventing movement. A drip used to encourage contractions will contain Syntocinon which is synthetic oxytocin. Oxytocin is another hormone produced naturally during labour. The amount of Syntocinon will be gradually increased until the contractions are coming regularly every 2-3 minutes. The rate of the drip can be altered depending on the response of the uterus and on your ability to cope with contractions; the idea is that you continue to progress in labour and if you need anything for pain relief then this can be arranged.

Monitoring in Labour

The strength and duration of contractions can be felt by resting a hand on your abdomen. The baby's heart rate can be checked from time to time with a fetal stethoscope or a Sonicaid machine. The Sonicaid uses ultrasound to pick up the movement of the baby's heart beating and converts this to audible sound.

If a continuous check of the baby's heart rate is required then a metal disc can be strapped to your abdomen which works on the same ultrasonic principle. Another metal disc can be strapped to your abdomen to record the contractions. Wires from the discs go to a machine beside you which transfers information received onto a continuous paper trace.

Once the waters are broken, it is possible to attach a small metal clip (fetal scalp electrode) to the baby's scalp. This is done during an internal examination perhaps after artificial rupture of the membranes, especially if there is meconium in the fluid. Wires from the metal clip go to a plastic disc strapped to your thigh and then to the machine. Some hospitals put a fine plastic tube up beside the baby's head once the waters have broken to measure the contractions.

Telemetry is a means of continuously monitoring the baby's heart rate using a fetal scalp electrode and a system of radio waves. This allows you to move about as you are not wired to

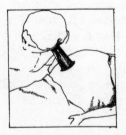

Monitoring the baby's heart rate with a fetal stethoscope

the machine that is recording. This is a new development and is not yet widely available. If the heart rate pattern suggests that the baby is lacking oxygen, this can be checked by sampling blood from the baby's scalp.

Fetal Blood Sampling

This involves the mother being either on her side with her upper leg supported by an assistant, or else in the lithotomy position. The doctor washes his/her hands thoroughly and puts on a sterile gown and gloves, then swabs your perineum with antiseptic solution. A hollow metal cone is then gently slipped into the vagina so that at the end of the cone, part of the baby's scalp can be seen. This is then sprayed with local anaesthetic and pricked so that a small blob of blood flows which can be sucked into a fine glass tube. This minute specimen is then taken for immediate testing to see if the baby is lacking oxygen and its blood is too acid.

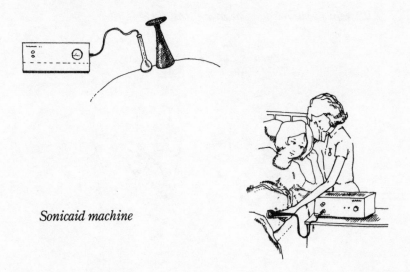

Sonicaid machine

Caesarean Birth

The history of Caesarean birth

The origin of Caesarean section is lost in ancient mythology. The word caesarean probably comes from the Latin 'caedere', meaning to cut. The operation was performed long before Julius Caesar was born, and contrary to popular belief it seems unlikely that he was delivered in this way as his mother was alive during the years of his campaigns. Originally the operation was performed on dead or dying mothers to save the baby, and it is only in the last 100 years that techniques have been developed so that the mother can survive a Caesarean section. As antiseptic, anaesthetic and surgical techniques have advanced so Caesarean birth has become safer, and the incidence of Caesarean births has increased, but it is still safer to have your baby normally. The maternal mortality rate is about 1 in 10,000 for all births but about 8 in 10,000 for Caesarean births.

Alternative positions for Caesarean scar

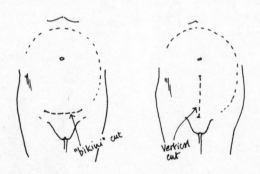

What Happens

The Caesarean operation

The operation involves opening the mother's abdomen either horizontally (the bikini cut) or vertically; both cuts are about 5"-6" long. The uterus lies in the middle with bowels above and behind. The bladder lies over the lower part of the uterus and has to be pushed down to get at the thinner lower segment of the uterus. The lower segment is then opened horizontally and the baby delivered through this false opening, followed by the placenta and membranes.

Then begins the longer process of putting the layers back together again. It may take only 5-10 minutes to deliver the baby but another 30-40 minutes to put the layers back together. The final skin layer can be closed by a hidden stitch which dissolves slowly and does not need to be removed, or with clips or external stitches which need to be removed 4-7 days later. Sometimes the doctor will drain any blood that might collect in the wound with a small plastic drain coming from the side of the wound and draining into a small glass bottle. The drain will be removed 1-2 days after the operation. The wound is covered either by spraying on a plastic protective layer, or with gauze and Elastoplast or similar sticky tape.

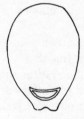 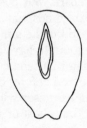

Possible sites of incision:
a) lower segment uterine incision
b) classical uterine incision

Coping with Caesarean

Very occasionally a vertical incision is made in the thicker more muscular upper segment of the uterus; this is called a classical Caesarean section, and may be necessary if, for example, there is a large fibroid in the lower segment. The modern lower segment Caesarean section gives a stronger scar that heals better and should withstand any future labour contractions. It is therefore important to know the type of scar you have in your uterus.

Note: A vertical scar on your abdomen does not necessarily mean a vertical scar in your uterus, which will usually be a horizontal lower segment scar.

Elective Caesarean Birth

An Elective Caesarean is one that is planned in advance before the mother goes into labour.

If you know you are going to have a Caesarean birth, then ask the doctors and midwives the whys and wherefores of the procedure before you come into hospital. You may like to talk to an anaesthetist about the choice of anaesthetic. If you know someone who has had a Caesarean section, perhaps she can give you some hints for coping with the post-natal period in hospital and later at home. In some areas there are support groups for women giving birth by Caesarean (see Page 102).

It is still important to prepare your body and mind. The relaxation exercises you learn in hospital antenatal classes or NCT classes will therefore still be helpful.

Once you know you are going to have a Caesarean you may feel unhappy about continuing to attend classes, but the relaxation will certainly help you before, during and after the Caesarean and the breathing exercises will help you afterwards with coughing and clearing your chest of secretions. For your sake and the baby's, if you are a smoker—STOP. It is also helpful to discuss your forthcoming Caesarean birth with the class; it may help answer some of your questions and may also unknowingly prepare someone else who may need an emergency Caesarean.

You will probably be admitted to hospital the night before your operation. It is worthwhile exploring your environment that evening, especially the ward that you will go to after the Caesarean. Make friends with the nurses, find the toilets, and try to foresee any problems that may lie ahead for you in the layout of the ward and your forthcoming limited mobility.

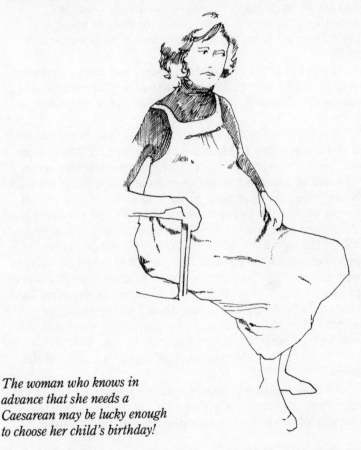

The woman who knows in advance that she needs a Caesarean may be lucky enough to choose her child's birthday!

Coping with Caesarean

A junior doctor will come to talk to you and examine you. He/she will then ask you to sign a form giving your consent to the operation. You will also see the doctor who will perform the operation; this could be your Consultant or his Registrar. This is an excellent opportunity to make sure you understand why the operation is necessary, how it will be done, who will be present and what type of anaesthetic you will have. The anaesthetist will also probably come to see you to make sure you are fit for anaesthetic and again discuss the type of anaesthetic planned. Be sure to tell the doctors about any tablets you are taking or any medicines to which you react badly.

If you are afraid of hospitals, or feel you cannot express your feelings easily to doctors, make sure your partner, a parent or a friend stays to help you find out all you want to know.

Before the operation a blood sample will be taken to check if you are anaemic and to cross-match blood for you in case you need a blood transfusion during or after the Caesarean. You will be asked not to eat or drink anything for at least six hours before the operation. Some hospitals will give you an enema so that the bowel is empty and does not get in the way. Your pubic hair will be shaved because the cut is usually made just at the top of the pubic hair line. You will be dressed in a practical but not very glamorous gown and your hair covered with a paper cap. You may be asked to drink a small quantity of antacid liquid to neutralise any acid in your stomach. This acid could be dangerous if you are sick either during or directly after the operation. In a drowsy state you could accidentally breathe the acid from the back of your throat into your lungs: if the acid is neutralised it is less irritant to the lungs.

All nail varnish and make-up must be removed before the operation, so that the colour of your lips and nails can be properly observed by the anaesthetist. For safety's sake, jewellery should also be removed, but your wedding ring can be taped over rather than removed if you prefer.

Some hospitals will give you an injection (pre-medication) before you go to theatre: this will make your mouth dry. You will not be given an injection to make you sleepy as this would also make the baby sleepy. The bladder must be empty before the operation or it will get in the way and could be accidentally damaged. A small plastic or rubber tube (a catheter) is put into the bladder to make sure it is empty. This may be done on the ward or when you are in theatre, either awake or asleep. If you are awake when this is done, practise your relaxation, open your legs and release any tension in the muscles around your vagina: this will make it easier for the nurse and therefore easier for you.

You will need a drip to give you fluid through a vein in your arm. The drip may be put up by a doctor on the ward or by the anaesthetist in theatre (see Page 44). Usually the fluid is a clear salty or sugary solution but later you may need a blood transfusion. Before you leave the ward and again in theatre you will have your pulse and blood pressure checked and the midwife will listen to the baby's heart beat.

A special cardiogram is used nowadays for both epidural and general anaesthetic section, so before the operation begins, the anaesthetist places three adhesive discs on your chest and attaches leads to them so that your heartrate can be continuously monitored.

Emergency Caesarean Birth

An Emergency Caesarean is usually performed during labour where either the mother's or baby's life is at risk. The preparations for an Emergency Caesarean birth are much the same as for an elective, but everything happens faster, which can be frightening. You will probably be asked to lie on your left side; this shifts the weight of the uterus away from the big

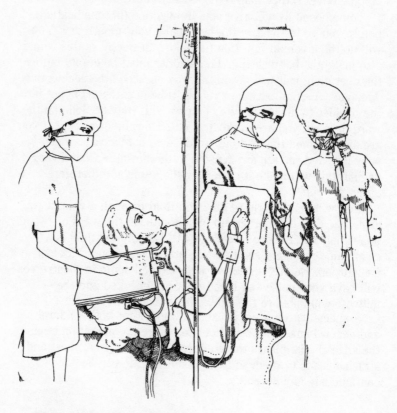

The operator and assistant are working beyond the drapes, while the anaesthetist monitors the mother's vital functions

blood vessels. You may also be given oxygen to breathe through a mask; both are ways of helping give the baby more oxygen.

Usually there is still time for the doctor to explain why you need a Caesarean. At times like this your partner can be very supportive. He will be nervous as well, but may understand what the doctor is saying better than you, especially if you have had pain-killing drugs and are drowsy. It is worthwhile one or other of you making sure you know the name of the doctor, so you can talk about the birth afterwards. Do not leave the hospital confused about why you needed a Caesarean and what to expect in future labours. You may need it explained several times.

It often helps to write down questions before the doctor comes, because he/she may appear to be so busy that all your questions are forgotten in the rush. It is very important for your feelings about yourself as a new mother, and your feelings about your baby, that you really understand what happened. If you were asleep for the birth, then do ask someone who was there to describe events; this will help you to build up a very precious picture of the first moments of your baby's life. Perhaps someone could take a photograph of the baby at, or soon after, birth. A Polaroid camera is ideal for this.

Choice of Anaesthetic

General Anaesthetic. This means that you are asleep for the operation. It may be necessary for an emergency Caesarean, or you may prefer the idea of being asleep. It is common practice to take you into the operating theatre and position you on the operating table before you are asleep. While the anaesthetist is checking equipment he will ask you to breathe oxygen through a mask. This will help your baby; it will not make you sleepy.

Next follows what is called the induction of the anaesthetic;

this means putting you off to sleep. It is the same as with any other anaesthetic, but with one very important addition. You will remember that we talked about neutralising the acid in your stomach.

An extra precaution is always taken at this stage to prevent acid stomach contents reaching the lungs at the moment of induction. As you go off to sleep an assistant will place fingers on your neck, pressing in a special way. This can be uncomfortable, but it is necessary for safety. You will be put to sleep by an injection given through the drip in your arm. This drug passes into your bloodstream and you fall asleep in about 30 seconds. The anaesthetist then gives you another injection which relaxes all your muscles. Once this has taken effect a tube is passed over the back of your throat and into your windpipe. When this is in place the assistant's pressure on your neck is released. The tube is then attached to a machine (ventilator) which breathes for you during the operation, and administers the right amount of gases to keep you asleep.

It usually takes 5-10 minutes to deliver the baby from your uterus; during this period you have a light anaesthetic so that the baby is not born too drowsy. Because of this, women occasionally have an awareness of voices or things happening; this can be disturbing, but the knowledge that it is for the baby's sake makes it easier to cope with; there will be no sensation of pain.

Once the baby is delivered the anaesthetist increases the amount of anaesthetic, and you stay deeply asleep while the obstetrician closes the layers in your abdomen. This will take 30-40 minutes.

It is worth telling the doctors before the operation that you would like to see your baby as soon as you wake up. This should ensure that the baby is kept warm in theatre ready to greet you and not rushed off to be washed and weighed. Inside the theatre there will be a special machine (a resuscitaire) used by paediatricians for checking newborn babies and giving them extra oxygen to breathe if they are sleepy. There may be an incubator for keeping the baby warm, which can also be used to transport the baby back to the postnatal ward; this does not necessarily mean that the baby has problems and will need to stay in an incubator once it gets to the ward. A more pleasant way of keeping your baby warm is for your partner to give it a cuddle and get to know the baby; later, on the way back to the ward, your baby could be kept warm next to you in the bed or on the trolley.

If the baby has been slow to breathe and is needing extra help, then it will be taken away by the paediatrician to the Special Care Baby Unit (see Page 80). Some doctors will allow partners into theatres even if the mother is having a general anaesthetic and then the moment of birth is witnessed by one of the parents. However, this is still a rare occurrence.

As you wake up and begin to be aware of the world again you will be turned onto your side, and saliva sucked out of your mouth before the tube in your throat is removed. As the tube is removed you may cough or occasionally vomit. You will then be moved from the operating table to a theatre trolley or into your own bed. You will be awake but sleepy within 2-3 minutes of the operation finishing.

A word of advice to the partner (this could equally apply to a parent or friend). If you are left waiting outside, this can be a very lonely and worrying time. You may want to be alone, or you might find it easier to phone someone else to come and be with you. It can take well over an hour from the time the mother leaves the labour room until she comes back to the ward so do not be alarmed at the length of time; it does not mean that a disaster has occurred. It would also be worthwhile asking if you could see, cuddle and get to know the baby during the time the mother is being stitched up. You could also be there to give her the baby when she wakes up. It can be a very moving experience to see a drowsy smile as her hand (drip and all) stretches out to touch and explore the new life.

Coping with Caesarean

Caesarean Birth with Epidural

Inside the operating theatre you will be lying on the table, literally the centre of attention. A blood pressure cuff will be placed on one arm; the drip is already in the other. A soft metal diathermy plate is strapped around one leg; the diathermy equipment is used to burn small blood vessels in the wound and thus control bleeding.

It may be difficult to recognise people in theatre dress, but you will soon recognise their voices. The atmosphere in theatre during a Caesarean is usually very happy and everyone will be keen to reassure you and boost your morale.

There are usually four doctors present: the anaesthetist, the obstetrician (who performs the operation), the assistant, and the paediatrician (who will check your baby after birth). There will be several nurses with different responsibilities. The two main nurses will be the scrub nurse, who is in charge of handing instruments to the operator, and your midwife. In teaching hospitals there may be students too.

You will also notice the resuscitaire, a special machine equipped with everything a paediatrician may need to help a newborn baby breathe properly. There may also be an incubator or a cot for the baby (see Page 47). The anaesthetist will be at your head, with your partner if he is to be with you. Next to the anaesthetist will be the anaesthetic machine. The scrub nurse will be close to your feet and next to her will be the instrument trolley.

Above you will be large circular theatre lights; sometimes a mirror can be arranged if you wish to see the operation.

With an epidural anaesthetic you will be aware of touch but not of pain and the operation will not start until the anaesthetist is happy that the epidural is effective. He/she will test you with a sharp needle or a very cold spray over your abdomen. Once the sensations of pain and cold have gone the epidural is working.

What Happens

The Operation

First of all the scrub nurse, operator and assistant wash their hands thoroughly and put on sterile gowns and gloves. Then everyone is ready to begin. Your abdomen is exposed and the doctor will clean your skin with a special antiseptic lotion. Then sterile towels will be draped over you, leaving only a small opening through which the operation will be performed. Unless you really want to see, the towels are placed in such a way as to provide a barrier.

It usually takes 5-10 minutes to get the baby out. During this time you may be aware of pushing and pulling, but not pain. The operating doctor will usually chat to you so that you know what stage he/she has reached. You may also hear a buzzing noise from time to time; this is the doctor using the diathermy machine.

When it comes to actually getting the baby out, the doctor's hand reaches deep into the uterus. This sensation can be very strange, as though the uterus is a deep handbag and the doctor is rummaging around to find something. If the baby is coming head first the doctor may be able to cup a hand under the head and lift it through the wound but sometimes small forceps are used instead. Once the head is through, the rest of the baby's body slips through easily in a similar fashion to a vaginal birth.

The operator's hand is passed into the uterus to lift the baby's head

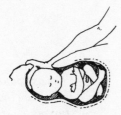

Coping with Caesarean

You may be asked to help by pushing or you may be aware of the assistant gently pushing on the top of your abdomen. When the baby is coming bottom first the bottom and legs are eased out first (the baby often passes water and meconium at this stage). Then the arms and finally the head come through the wound—the process is similar to a vaginal breech birth (see Page 61).

The next moment is one of great relief and joy. The baby is born; it usually splutters, gasps and may cry. The umbilical cord is clamped and cut and the new life begins to exist separately from you. As soon as possible the baby will be given back to you, to see, to touch, to smell and to cuddle. The paediatrician may want to check the baby first and suck out any fluid from its nose and mouth. Should there be a delay in the baby breathing the paediatrician will give the baby more oxygen, and sometimes may need to pass a tube into the baby's lungs.

Meanwhile the doctor delivers the placenta and membranes

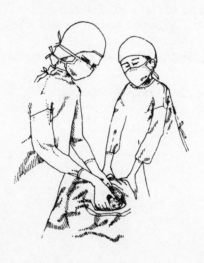

The assistant presses on the fundus to help the baby out

and begins to close up the wound. This next bit may take about 30-40 minutes, which can be rather tedious, and sometimes you may feel sick. After you and the baby have spent some time saying hello to one another you may feel you would like a rest and the anaesthetist will give you something to help you relax or to relieve the sickness. However, you may feel fantastic and enjoy every moment with your baby. While the surgery continues, you may be able to breast-feed; the skin-to-skin contact will feel good even if the position is not ideal for successful feeding.

Occasionally the epidural is less effective and you feel pain. If this gets unpleasant then the best thing is to have a general anaesthetic and this can be arranged by the anaesthetist whenever you want it.

Once the operation is finished, the towels will be removed and you are cleaned up. There may appear to be a lot of blood, but this is blood mixed with fluid, so it tends to look worse.

After the operation you will be transferred to your bed or a

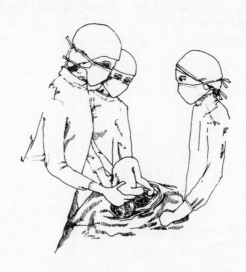

*The baby is
lifted out*

trolley. It is rather exciting to go back to the postnatal ward with your baby warmly wrapped up and snuggled next to you, so if this doesn't happen automatically why not ask for the baby yourself?

Local Anaesthetic

Sometimes the epidural anaesthetic fails to work, and if you wish to be awake during the birth of your baby by Caesarean it may be possible for the obstetrician to use a local anaesthetic. In this case a fairly large amount of weak local anaesthetic is injected into the skin of the abdomen, and then into the muscles and peritoneum underneath. Pain from cutting is blocked, but some sensation of pulling and stretching remains and the delivery of the head through the cut in the uterus may be quite uncomfortable, rather like the stretching of the vaginal opening in a normal birth.

Few younger doctors, unless they have worked in developing countries, will have had practice in this method, but you could ask your obstetrician if he/she has had experience with this technique. As with epidural anaesthetic, if you find it unpleasant then a general anaesthetic can still be given.

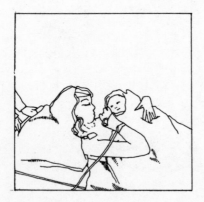

Going back to the ward with the baby on the trolley

What Happens

Forceps and Ventouse Delivery

The History of Forceps and Ventouse

Forceps were invented in England in the late 16th century by a Huguenot doctor called Peter Chamberlen, and have been modified by various obstetricians over the course of 300 years. They are used to pull, or turn and pull, the baby's head through the birth canal. The smallest type are called Wriggley's forceps; they are protective and pulling forceps. Those used most frequently for pulling are larger and are called Simpson's or Neville Barnes forceps. When turning and pulling forceps are needed, then Kielland's forceps are used.

In 1953 Malstrom invented an alternative instrument called a ventouse (or vacuum extractor) which works on a suction principle and can be used to pull, or turn and pull, the baby through the birth canal. The ventouse has the added advantage that it can be used safely late in the first stage, before the cervix is fully dilated.

Forceps Delivery

Forceps come in two halves which lock together. Each has a blade which cups around the baby's head, and handles to pull on. There are different lengths and shapes of forceps for use in different circumstances. The smallest, called Wriggley's forceps, are useful at the time of a Caesarean birth; sometimes they are used to protect the soft skull-bones of a premature infant. Similar protection can be given by larger forceps to the aftercoming head of a breech birth. The larger forceps such as Simpson's are used for pulling if the baby is in the anterior position; Kielland's forceps are used for turning and then pulling if the baby is in the posterior or transverse position.

When the decision has been made to use forceps the mother will need good pain relief, especially if it is necessary to turn

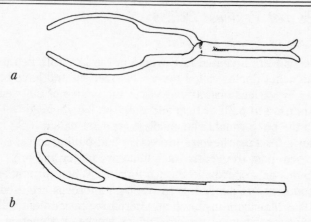

a

b

The forceps blades have two curves:
a) the cephalic curve, designed to fit the baby's head
b) the pelvic curve, designed so that the blades fit in with the
curve of the birth canal

the baby's head before the delivery. A general anaesthetic, an epidural or a caudal anaesthetic (all of which are the province of an anaesthetist or specially trained obstetrician) will be used. A caudal anaesthetic is similar to the epidural, except that the epidural space is approached lower down, near your tailbone. This can be used to give one injection of local anaesthetic to numb your vagina and vulva for a forceps delivery. More often the obstetrician will use a local anaesthetic called a pudendal block.

It is common nowadays for partners to be allowed to remain for forceps deliveries, except sometimes for those performed under general anaesthetic. You will be positioned with your legs up in stirrups. This is called the lithotomy position. It is helpful if your shoulders are still propped up, both because you can then assist the doctor by pushing better and also because it helps you to see the baby. The doctor puts on a plastic apron, sterile gown and gloves, cleans your vulva with antiseptic and puts sterile sheets over your legs and abdomen. Often the doctor will pass a catheter and empty the bladder at this stage. The doctor will then examine you again to assess the position of the baby and to make sure there is enough room for the baby to come through.

If you do not have an epidural or general anaesthetic you may find that Entonox helps you to cope with this necessary but thorough and sometimes uncomfortable examination.

Then the pudendal block will be given. During the examination the doctor finds two bony points in your pelvis: the nerve which carries sensations from the vagina runs close to these points, so it is here that local anaesthetic is injected. He will also inject local anaesthetic directly into the vaginal entrance to make sure it is numb before cutting the skin, if the opening needs to be made bigger (episiotomy)—this is usually, but not always, necessary.

The forceps are then inserted, first one half and then the other, so that the blades cup around the baby's head and the handles lock together outside. If the baby's head needs to be turned this will be done first; once the baby is lying the right

a) Mid cavity forceps delivery. The forceps blades cup aroung the baby's head as it nestles within the cavity of the pelvis

b) The forceps have brought the baby's head down onto the perineum and the baby's head is about to crown

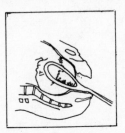
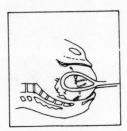

way round the doctor and you work together, so that with each contraction, you push and the doctor pulls. Once the baby's head has come through, the forceps are removed and you can peer through your legs to see and touch the baby's head and, with the help of the doctor, deliver the baby up onto your abdomen. A paediatrician may need to check your baby soon after delivery and perhaps give it some help with breathing, so after the cord had been clamped and cut you may have to part with the baby temporarily. It is helpful if the resuscitaire is placed so that you can still see your baby.

The placenta and membranes are delivered next, and you may be given an injection in your leg as the baby is being born to help speed up the process and avoid too much bleeding. All that remains is for the doctor to stitch up the episiotomy and then bliss—you can have your legs down and really cuddle your new baby; skin-to-skin contact and breast feeding at this time can be very rewarding. The baby may have a long head and some bruises on its face after a forceps delivery, but these go away over the next 24-48 hours.

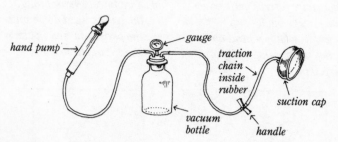

Vacuum extractor (Ventouse)

What Happens

Ventouse Delivery

The ventouse has a similar function to the forceps, and can be used to turn and deliver the baby. The preparation and choice of pain relief are also similar. When everything is ready the doctor checks the baby's position and applies a metal cup about 6 cm in diameter to the baby's head. Tubing comes from the cup to a special suction bottle placed close to the obstetrician, and a helper creates the suction by using a pump which is like a reverse bicycle pump. When the correct negative pressure has been reached, which takes 5-10 minutes, doctor and mother work together, pulling and pushing respectively with each contraction. Two or three contractions should bring success. After a ventouse delivery the baby will have an especially long head. This is called a chignon (meaning a bun in French). Although it may look alarming, it is quite harmless and will settle down over 24-48 hours.

As stated previously, the ventouse can sometimes be used late in the first stage of labour before the cervix is fully open. Apart from this, the different types of forceps and the ventouse are interchangeable. Obstetricians are trained to be safe and efficient with both forceps and ventouse but they will usually develop their own preferences for coping with specific situations.

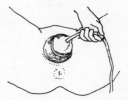

Delivery by vacuum extractor

Episiotomy

The area between the opening of your vagina and your back passage (perineum) is numbed with local anaesthetic injected between contractions. Once the anaesthetic is effective, a cut can be made during a contraction when the perineum is being stretched. This cut is 1"-2" long, usually on the right side.

This cut widens the opening of the vagina and the baby's head will soon be born.

To repair an episiotomy or tear, your legs will be placed in stirrups in the lithotomy position and more local anaesthetic injected into the wound so you do not feel the stitches. There are three layers to be stitched, first the lining of the vagina, then the muscle layer, then the outside skin layer. Usually the material used will dissolve in the next ten days and you will heal in four to six weeks, but the tenderness may take longer to go away.

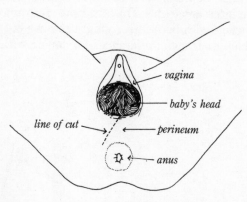

Episiotomy cut

4 Premature Births, Breech Births and Multiple Births

Let us consider the special problems of the baby that is born too early, the baby that is bottom (breech) first and multiple births where there are two or more babies. The reason why premature labour occurs is often not known but it is more common with abnormalities in the shape of the uterus; a weak cervix which may follow a previous termination of pregnancy or operation to the cervix (see Page 27); a uterus that is overstretched, for example by twins; or a uterus made irritable by a placental abruption (see Page 27).

Premature Births

A baby born after 26 weeks of pregnancy may survive with today's intensive neonatal care (neonatal means newborn). A baby is said to be premature if it is born before the end of 37 completed weeks of pregnancy; at 26 weeks the survival rate is about 10%, rising to 50% at 28 weeks and almost 100% by 34 weeks. (These figures vary from unit to unit.) There are many problems with very premature babies because everything is immature, but the main problem is with the lungs. Up to 34 weeks it is common for the premature baby to need assistance with breathing, which may mean using a mechanical ventilator or just increasing the amount of oxygen in the air it breathes.

If you think you are in labour prematurely, you must go directly to hospital. It is sometimes possible to stop premature labour with drugs given through a drip. These drugs belong to a family of drugs called sympathomimetics which means they have a similar effect on your body to the natural response to fear; therefore when you have a drip to stop premature labour you may feel your heart beating rapidly and find you are trembling, as well as the desired effect which is to stop the uterus contracting. If the hospital you go to does not have a neonatal unit that can cope with very small babies you may be transferred by ambulance to a bigger hospital. It is not always possible to stop a premature labour, or even delay it, especially if your waters have broken.

A premature baby is smaller and more delicate, so its birth needs to be gentle. The premature baby's head is particularly vulnerable. If a premature baby is coming head first then it can be delivered safely through the vagina. Sometimes a doctor will recommend an epidural so that the strong urge to push is removed, and the action of the uterus contracting and more controlled pushing will deliver the baby more slowly. If the muscles of the perineum (see Page 58) are thick and rigid, especially if this is a first baby, then the doctor or midwife will perform an episiotomy to prevent any undue pressure on the soft head. In second and subsequent babies, the muscles tend to be less rigid and an episiotomy is not always required. Sometimes small forceps are used to cup around and protect the baby's head (see Page 53).

Up to 34 weeks of pregnancy there is a lot of liquor (water) around the baby, so the baby is free to move and change its position frequently. It is therefore not uncommon for a premature baby to come bottom first. In such cases, observation has shown that from 28-32 weeks the chances of survival may be less if the baby is born through the vagina. This is because the vulnerable baby's head is the last part to come through the birth canal and may get caught by the cervix if the smaller body has slipped through before it is fully open. Under these circumstances, a Caesarean section may be the safest way of delivering the baby, but each case must be considered individually.

A paediatrician will always be present for the birth of a premature baby and will explain to you what is happening and why. You may be able to see or hold the baby briefly before it goes to the Special Care Baby Unit (see Page 80).

Difficult Births

Breech Births

The most common cause of a baby coming breech first is prematurity, but 3-4% of mature babies still come breech first. Usually the cause is unknown but it may be due to an abnormal shape of the mother's uterus or something blocking the opening to the pelvis such as a fibroid, an ovarian cyst or a low-lying placenta. There may be an excess amount of liquor after 34 weeks so that the baby remains mobile. The stretchy uterus of a woman who has had several babies also allows the baby more mobility. The problem may be with the baby; an abnormal baby may come breech first and in multiple births one of the babies may be breech first.

There are various kinds of breech presentation. Sometimes the baby's feet are curled up beneath the breech, sometimes it is sitting crosslegged with the knees bent and sometimes the knees are straight with the baby's feet beside its head. The first position means that the breech does not fit snugly into the mother's bony pelvis and when the waters break the cord can sometimes slip past the baby's bottom; this is called a cord prolapse (see Page 29). If this happens the baby must be born by an Emergency Caesarean.

When an obstetrician finds that there is a breech presentation after 34 weeks of pregnancy, then he/she may try to turn the baby to come head first. This cannot always be done, if for example there is a scar in the uterus or there has been any bleeding from the placenta during pregnancy. Some doctors prefer not to try and turn a baby; many will turn themselves anyway, and those that are turned frequently turn back again!

You may be able to help the baby turn itself by relaxing each day for 30-60 minutes either in the kow-tow position or lying on your back on the floor with a pillow under your bottom and your legs stretched up the wall. Either position helps the baby's bottom to come out of the pelvis and then to turn around if it wants to. If you feel it turn, stand up quickly!

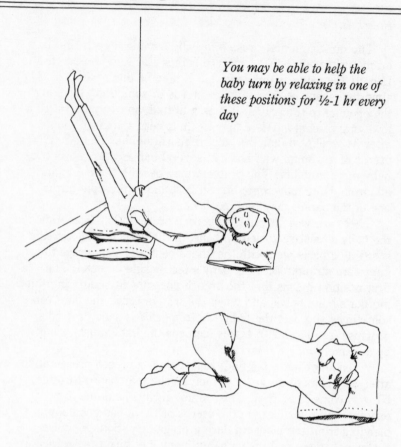

You may be able to help the baby turn by relaxing in one of these positions for ½-1 hr every day

In the same way that obstetricians agree to differ about turning breech babies, they also disagree about methods of delivery. Some favour Caesarean section for all cases, while others recommend a more conservative 'wait and see' approach; if the baby comes down the birth canal normally during labour then they proceed to a vaginal breech birth, but if the baby sticks at any stage an Emergency Caesarean is performed. When considering the right method of birth other

Difficult Births

problems are taken into consideration and if there is a second factor such as high blood pressure then it may be considered safer to deliver the baby by an Elective Caesarean.

If you are planning for a vaginal breech delivery then the size of the baby, especially the head, will be assessed by the doctor feeling it through your abdomen and then getting more exact measurements with ultrasound. The size of your bony pelvis is also checked by the doctor who is particularly feeling for any prominent bones sticking into the birth canal and then direct measurements are taken by X-raying your pelvis. This is called pelvimetry. The main anxiety with a vaginal breech birth is the baby's head which comes last through the birth canal and does not have time to shape itself (mould) to the mother's pelvis, as happens when a baby is born head first.

Vaginal Breech Birth

You may be advised to have an epidural for your labour. In the second stage the doctor may need to help the baby's legs and body out of the vagina, using forceps to protect and guide the head over the perineum, so good pain relief is helpful and you will be more relaxed. Also, if you do not open up and a Caesarean is necessary, then you can have this done with an epidural anaesthetic. However, many obstetricians (and mothers) prefer a breech birth without an epidural. A compromise can be for the anaesthetist to put the epidural catheter in place early in labour but for no local anaesthetic to be injected unless it is needed.

The first stage of labour is similar to normal labour. In the second stage the baby's bottom comes down the birth canal and stretches the perineum in the same way as the head. At this stage you will be helped into the lithotomy position. Unless the perineum is very soft and stretchy the doctor will inject local anaesthetic and perform an episiotomy to give the baby plenty of room. As the baby's bottom emerges you can tell its sex; at this stage it frequently passes water and meconium. It can be exciting to watch all this happen in a mirror if you can get a nurse to hold one in the right position for you and make sure your shoulders are well propped up.

Sometimes your pushing alone will deliver the baby as far as its armpits; if not, the doctor helps the legs to come out and then carefully brings out a length of umbilical cord so that the cord is loose and not stretched. Then the baby's arms are helped out; to do this the doctor may turn the baby's body from side to side so that each arm can slip out easily underneath the arch of your pubic bone. If you can see what is happening then the baby is frequently wriggling at this stage with its head still inside the vagina. It is left to hang so that the weight of its own body helps the head to come down.

The baby's legs are then lifted up and supported by an assistant while the doctor places forceps around the baby's head to protect it and deliver it slowly and in a controlled fashion. If the birth of the unmoulded head is too quick then the soft tissues inside the baby's skull may tear and the baby may be handicapped. If there is insufficient time to put on forceps, the doctor can slow and control the birth of the head with a special technique using his hands only.

Multiple Births

The incidence of twins is about 1 in 80 births in the UK and the incidence of triplets about 1 in 6,000. Twins are usually non-identical (two separate eggs fertilised by two separate sperms and developed together) but sometimes twins are identical, which means that they have developed from one egg and one sperm. Non-identical twins, triplets and other multiple births are now more common because of fertility drugs, which can cause a woman to release more than one egg each month.

With multiple pregnancies the mother may be very

Difficult Births

uncomfortable because of the size of the uterus. She also tends to be tired and anaemic because the babies use up all her stores of iron and vitamins. This can be counteracted by taking extra iron and vitamins during the pregnancy. There is also an increased tendency to develop high blood pressure and the mother may well go into labour prematurely if the uterus is overstretched. It is not uncommon for one of the babies to come breech first or even to lie sideways in the uterus.

Triplets are usually delivered by Elective Caesarean section; twins are usually safe to be born vaginally, but if one is coming breech first then all the precautions need to be taken as previously described. The second twin is particularly at risk and the doctor may well need to help with forceps or ventouse. Some obstetricians will advise an epidural anaesthetic for twins, especially if one of the twins is coming breech first.

After the birth there may be the added concern of the babies being in the Special Care Unit if they are premature or if the birth has been particularly difficult. Then there are problems with feeding. Twins can still be breast-fed with one on each breast and with their bodies resting on pillows and tucked under the mother's arms. At home there can be extra problems with getting two (or more) of everything and needing extra time to manage the babies. A social worker may be able to help provide a home help in the early days and to advise if there are financial problems. You could also contact other mothers with twins (see address on Page 102).

5 After the Birth

Pain Relief

The method used for pain relief depends on whether you had an epidural or general anaesthetic. Sometimes the epidural is left in for a short period and further top-ups are given for pain relief; if the epidural has been removed or if you had a general anaesthetic then pain and sickness (if you feel this) are eased by giving injections into your bottom or thigh.

In the first 24 hours after the birth you need regular shots to relieve the pain; this helps you to cope with coughing, passing urine and moving. Once you are drinking, you can change from injections to pain-relieving tablets. Some hospitals concoct their own special mixtures, usually with a soluble pain-killer plus peppermint water for wind and an antacid for heartburn.

All the pain-relieving drugs are safe for breast-feeding mothers to take. The amounts passing to the baby in the milk will be negligible. It is therefore better to have adequate relief from pain and discomfort than to try to manage without tablets or injections.

Passing Urine

Some hospitals leave a catheter in place for the first night. Otherwise you have to learn to use a bedpan. It may be better to get the nurses to help you sit out on a commode or ask them to put the bedpan on the edge of the bed so that you can sit on it with your legs over the edge; this is more like sitting on a toilet—so relax your pelvic floor muscles and let it flow. If you still have no success the nurses may help by passing a catheter to release the urine and then removing it again. After the first night it is worth while taking time and, with help, getting to a toilet.

After the Birth

Bowels

Your bowels are unlikely to open the first day, but you can
get wind pains, which may be particularly severe around the
second or third days. Suppositories or a gentle enema can help
to get the wind shifted. Do not try to hold wind back; bowel
problems are common after all deliveries so it is better to make
a joke about it. You may get piles after a Caesarean birth, and
if these become really painful special creams and suppositories
will help to shrink them and ease the discomfort. Ice packs can
also be very soothing. From the second day onwards it is
probably helpful to take a regular laxative at night so that your
motions are soft and you do not have to strain. Laxatives
which make the motions softer and bulkier are best if you are
breast-feeding. Bran is particularly helpful. Senokot should be
avoided if you are breast-feeding.

Fluids

You will probably keep the intravenous drip for 12-24 hours
after the birth. This will give your body its liquid requirements.
You will have mouth-washes and sips of water at first, and
then gradually build up the amounts you drink, especially if
you are feeling sick (retching with a fresh scar is not pleasant).
Avoid fizzy drinks; they can cause very strong wind pains.

Food

Once you are drinking freely you can start on solid foods,
building up from a light diet to a full meal as your body
dictates. Fruit and fruit juices will help your bowels, but do not
overdo it if you are breast-feeding or the baby may get
diarrhoea. Bran in your diet is preferable.

Coughing

It is important to cough and clear phlegm from your chest after an operation, especially if you have had a general anaesthetic. If you are a smoker the problem can be worse and you risk developing a chest infection. A physiotherapist will come to help you cough and inhalations may help to loosen the secretions. It is worth while making sure that you have some pain relief before your physiotherapy. The physiotherapist will teach you to support your scar with your hands when you cough; this is also helpful when you laugh or when going to the toilet.

Moving and Getting Up

During the first 24 hours after the birth, it is important to keep your legs moving in bed. In this way the circulation of blood in your legs is improved, which helps prevent clots forming in the veins in your legs. Some hospitals give you special support stockings to wear in bed for the same reason. If you are likely to get clots you may be given injections to help thin the blood until you are fully mobile.

Your bottom may feel stiff and sore at first and if so the nurses can give you a soft ring to sit on, but the sooner you can move and get out of bed the better.

To get out of bed you will need help from the nurses and physiotherapists to start with, first to sit out in a chair and then to get to the toilet and bathroom. After the first day or two you will be able to get up on your own; remember to go slowly and take your time. Do not be surprised at the length of time it takes to get out of bed and walk to the toilet, and if you feel uncertain make sure someone is with you. Try to walk upright as soon as possible—you are not about to burst open.

If your bed has pedals that raise and lower it, then keep the bed low so that it is easier to get in and out. It can help to have a 'monkey bar' overhead to help you pull yourself up in bed. To get yourself out of bed try lying on your back, then rolling onto your side; now gradually push yourself up into a sitting position, swinging your legs over the edge of the bed at the same time. From this position you can push yourself up to standing; a well-positioned chair to hang onto may help. The same procedure in reverse will help you get back into bed.

If your baby is in the special care unit, you can see it as soon as you can get into a wheelchair. The unit will give you a polaroid photo of your baby if you are unable to get there. Your partner will also be able to visit and keep you informed.

The Bell

Most hospitals have single rooms for mothers after a Caesarean birth. In this way you get plenty of rest and other mothers are not disturbed in the night by the extra attention given to you. However, the room can feel very lonely, and far from help. Make sure you know where the bell is and that it is in a position you can reach easily when you need to summon help. When you are left alone ask to have the cot close to your bed to begin with so you can soothe the baby; it is very frustrating to have the baby crying a few feet away from you, and when the ward is busy the nurse may not answer your bell immediately.

Sleep

To begin with you will be propped up in bed to sleep, and pain-killing injections will help. Later it is wise to have a tablet for pain relief before going to sleep; your sleep is very important and you do not want a few precious hours disturbed by pain.

The first night you will probably be left alone in your room, and the baby will be taken to the nursery. If you are wanting to breast-feed your baby, then make sure the night staff are aware of this fact, and they will only give the baby water or sugar water to drink. You may feel you need to rest the next night and ask for the baby to go to the nursery again. The nurses can always wake you and bring the baby to you for feeds, or you may feel ready to keep the baby with you overnight; if you do you will still need to summon help to get the baby out of the cot for the first couple of days because lifting is too painful for you.

Demand feeding can be exhausting in the early days even after a normal delivery; recovering from an operation *and* trying to respond positively to the baby every 2-3 hours throughout the night can be just too much, so do ask for more help or let the baby go back to the nursery for a while if you find it difficult to cope. Tiredness is partly responsible for the crying and feelings of being unable to cope which often come about the fourth day after the birth.

Later you will probably be moved into a bigger ward with other women and then it is not only *your* baby crying that will disturb you but *their* babies as well; it seems that just as you manage to get off to sleep, you are being woken at some unearthly hour for breakfast!

During the day you will have rest periods, so use every available second to relax and sleep. If you get desperate at night then a mild sleeping tablet such as chloral hydrate may help you sleep; this is safe to take if you are breast-feeding but you should avoid Valium or Mogadon, which can affect the baby.

Feeding the Baby

Breast-feeding is not only perfectly feasible after a Caesarean, it is to be recommended because it helps the uterus return to its normal size. You may be able to breast-feed straight away if you have had an epidural, or are not too drowsy after a general

Possible feeding positions

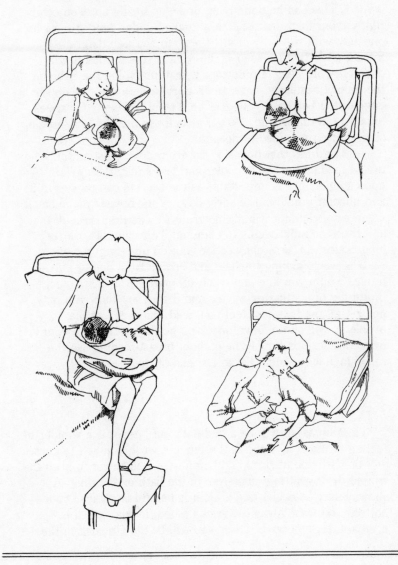

anaesthetic. To begin with you will need help positioning the baby so that it can suckle successfully without lying on your wound. This can be done lying down or sitting up. You can lie flat on your back with the baby tucked under your arm, or on one side with the baby cradled next to you (see diagrams). Sitting up in bed is easier if the back rest is in the upright position; then place a pillow on your tummy and the baby on the pillow. Similarly, you can sit upright on a chair or on the edge of the bed with your feet on a stool to keep your knees higher than the wound. Do not attempt to use the low 'nursing chairs' often provided in hospital.

A nightdress that opens at the front is very useful for breast-feeding (cotton is cooler and less sticky than nylon). A good support bra is important, as the breasts can be very full and uncomfortable in the early days. Your breasts make small volumes of rich nutritious colostrum for the first three days and then the milk begins to come in. This can take a little longer after a Caesarean section, but do not give up hope.

It is worth asking for help and advice from one or two nurses whom you like and trust; otherwise it is easy to get a multitude of conflicting advice and if they are busy you may not get all the help you feel you need, but many of the problems will settle down once you get home and into your own routine. For further help about breast-feeding see the recommended reading list at the end of the book.

Washing

The first wash will be a bed-bath but later it is a wonderful feeling to make it to the bathroom and wash yourself (a nurse will be with you at first). To begin with it is better to keep the wound dry by sitting on a stool in the bath or kneeling. A shower may be easier and a bidet is helpful to cleanse your bottom and wash away the sticky blood (lochia) which is normal after any birth. Later you will be able to soak in the

After the Birth

bath, wound and all, and washing your hair is a real morale-booster.

The Wound

It helps to wear knickers that come up to your waist (real passion killers!) rather than briefs where the elastic may chafe the wound. Similarly, avoid sanitary belts, which may rub. Sometimes the wound becomes infected and looks red and inflamed; this is quite painful, but the pain can be eased by a doctor or nurse draining the pus by making a small hole in the wound with a probe. A poultice or heat pad placed over the wound may also help draw the pus out. Salt added to your bath water is a good antiseptic to encourage healing. As the wound heals it may become very itchy; baby oil will help soften the scar and relieve the itching. It is not uncommon to feel numb around the scar; this feeling may last several months, and sometimes a small patch of skin may be permanently numb.

Sometimes a small plastic drain is used to drain away any blood that might collect under the skin into a small glass bottle. If you have a drain this will usually be removed the day after your operation by gently pulling it out. The sensation is one of a momentary aching discomfort rather than pain.

There are several ways of closing the skin layer; some stitches are hidden and dissolve so that there is nothing to remove later. Some stitches are hidden but do not dissolve; these are fixed at either end of the wound with a small bead and are easily removed by cutting one bead free and pulling the other, and thus the thread, out of the wound. Individual clips and stitches can be more painful and take longer to remove. If you are worried about this then ask for something to help relax you and relieve pain before the nurse starts.

Stitches in the 'bikini cut' are usually removed after 4-5 days, but with an up and down cut they will be left in for 7-10 days.

Coping with Caesarean

Bleeding from the Vagina (Lochia)

After the birth you will bleed like a period to start off with; this is called lochia. The lochia is red at first, but by about the fifth day it will be changing to be a brown colour and resemble the loss at the end of your period. It finally changes to a watery yellow-brown or pink discharge. Normal sanitary pads should be sufficient to cope with the bleeding but if you notice the bleeding becoming heavier or if you pass clots then you should tell the doctor, as this may indicate an infection in the uterus or that a piece of placenta or membrane is still inside the womb. This can be checked by ultrasound. If the check is positive then your uterus will be gently scraped under a general anaesthetic until it is empty.

Infections

After a Caesarean you may get an infection in your urine, chest, breasts, wound or uterus. If you have a persistent fever, the doctors will check you for any site of infection and you will need to take antibiotics. Antibiotics can make you feel rather tired; some of the penicillins may give you diarrhoea and also make the baby slightly loose if you are breast-feeding. The problem is unlikely to be so severe that you need to stop breast-feeding.

Visitors

For the first day, visiting will probably be limited to your partner only. After this it is sensible to restrict your visitors to close family and friends so you do not get too tired talking to everybody. If you have other children they will also be able to visit you and see the new baby. Some hospitals have special visiting times for children so it is worthwhile finding out the rules beforehand.

After the Birth

This can be a difficult time of separation from your partner and other children. Their visits will help bridge the gap but can also be distressing, especially answering such questions as 'why can't mummy come home today' when emotionally that is where you long to be. If it is your first baby, your partner can learn with you how to change and bath the baby when he comes to visit you. If you are bottle-feeding he can also learn about this and thus have more confidence to give you the help and support you will need at home.

Problems at Home

The longer you stay in hospital, the more disruptive it will be to your family, especially if it was not planned in advance. If there are problems at home then discuss them with a social worker, who may be able to arrange temporary help to see your family over the crisis.

Feelings

Immediately after the birth, the mother's feelings towards her new baby may vary from intense maternal love to indifference and unreality. Studies have shown that about 40% of mothers find that the elation and love for the baby they expected to feel immediately in fact takes several days to evolve. After a long and difficult birth, the mother frequently feels a sense of relief that it is all over; she may be delighted with the baby but her relief and tiredness are overriding and there is no room for other emotions.

Skin-to-skin and eye-to-eye contact are very helpful. A newborn baby's skin is delightfully soft and warm and as most delivery rooms are kept very warm it is safe for you to touch and explore your new baby from top to toe. If the baby has been wrapped up, undo the wrapping and see for yourself; explore the tiny fingers and toes, feel the limbs moving just as they used to move inside your body and study your baby's face. It is important to see that the baby is dry, especially the hair, because wet skin loses heat more quickly than dry. It is very rewarding to put the baby to the breast as soon as possible; this first attempt may not be an instant sucess, for the baby may be tired as well. It does, however, provide an excellent opportunity for the baby to smell, taste and feel you.

Many mothers also describe a time of getting to know their baby and appreciating him or her as a separate individual. It is hard to imagine that the baby that was inside the womb is now the baby in the cot. The baby in the womb was someone you could fantasise about, but this real little person is a stranger you have to get to know, just as the baby is also getting to know you from the outside.

It is common for depression (the 'blues') to set in about the third or fourth day after childbirth. The new mother may find herself crying and unable to explain why; she may be irritable, anxious, forgetful, confused and feel depersonalised; she may complain of headaches or fear rejection from her husband. She may express fears about the baby, that it is abnormal and no-one will tell her, or she may feel inadequate and unable to cope, and sometimes she may express negative feelings towards the baby.

There are many ways in which the 'blues' are manifested; the symptoms may only last a day but sometimes they can go on for a week or two. If there is a real problem, it is best to seek advice and help to overcome the depression.

Post-natal depression needs specialised psychiatric help and possibly even hospitalisation in special units for mother and baby. Depression can be more common after a Caesarean birth; not only is the body readjusting to changing hormone levels, but it is also coping with recovery from a major operation with physical discomfort, tiredness and possibly infection to compound the problems. It can be depressing to keep asking for help and relying on others to look after your baby when

After the Birth

other mothers seem to be managing alone. It can also be depressing to see women who had normal deliveries go home long before you; much as your spirit may be ready to be home, your body needs extra rest and nursing care because you have had an operation.

You may feel bad about feeling bad; after all, some helpful person may say, you have a live healthy baby, what more can you ask for? Depression is often a problem after an emergency Caesarean because the labour did not go according to your expectations, and you may have had fears that you or your baby were going to die. You may feel cheated of the experience of a vaginal delivery, for which you had been preparing all these months. You may feel you have failed and not performed as a 'real' woman would have done, and to prove it you think that your body is scarred and ugly. If you had a general anaesthetic you may have doubts about your baby; 'Is it really mine?' or even 'Did my baby die and is this a replacement baby?' You may feel angry with the baby for causing the pain and the difficult birth, and then feel guilty for even allowing such a thought to cross your mind.

This may all sound terribly pessimistic, but these are all feelings which have been expressed by mothers and it is important to express them and face them. This is why it is vital to understand the chain of events that lead to a Caesarean birth, and to realise that failure on your part does not come into it.

You need space and time to express your feelings and medical staff need the time and the empathy to pick up on your need to talk and to cry. Time, understanding and explanation are far more important than pills and well-meaning people saying 'pull yourself together'. Try to share your feelings with your partner. He will also have had fears of losing the two most important people in the world to him, and may welcome the chance to talk about the experience.

If you have no partner to help you, this can be a particularly difficult time. Parents and friends can provide a sensitive listening ear, or perhaps you may value the chance to talk to a social worker; she may be able to provide practical advice as well as emotional support. There are Caesarean section support groups in several parts of the UK and a mother who had a similar experience may be able to see you in hospital or at home. (See addresses on Page 102.)

Let us consider the problem of separation; how detrimental is this to the mother/child relationship in the long run? It does appear that the concept of bonding like glue—if mother and baby are instantly stuck together then all will be well—is far too simplistic. Separation problems are something the medical profession is now more aware of, and every effort is made to unite mother and baby as soon as possible. Parents are encouraged to visit their babies in the Special Care Baby Units and to touch them and help to care for them. Building up the relationship may take longer but with understanding and patience it will develop.

On the positive side, many mothers do feel completely compensated after a Caesarean by the end result of a beautiful healthy baby, and as they begin to heal and become more mobile so the joy of this new baby gives them a strength to recover more quickly than recovery from other forms of major surgery. It is then possible to look upon the Caesarean birth as a positive experience, and to say 'my baby was born a cut above'.

After a Difficult Vaginal Delivery

The main problems after a difficult vaginal birth are passing urine, opening your bowels and sitting down on your episiotomy scar. Sometimes you can be bruised and swollen, so that you need a catheter to pass urine for the first day or two. Passing urine into a warm bath may help if you are having trouble. Laxatives will help to keep your motions soft and less painful to pass. A soft pillow to sit on, or a rubber ring, can help for a painful episiotomy. Ice packs also help reduce the swelling. It is important to wash your bottom carefully after you have been to the toilet; most hospitals have bidets for this purpose. A little salt in your bath water encourages the episiotomy to heal. It is important to keep your bottom dry, as dampness around the wound encourages infection. A hair dryer can work wonders if you find drying with a towel very uncomfortable.

Usually the recovery period after a forceps or ventouse delivery is very similar to that for a normal delivery. You are soon able to do everything for yourself and your baby and will not be delayed from going home.

You may feel disappointment or a sense of failure that you did not push the baby out yourself, but again adequate explanations of the events that led up to you needing assistance, and being able to express your feelings, are important to help you come to terms with events.

You may fear damage to the vagina from the forceps or ventouse or from a larger episiotomy, but the vagina is like the inside of your mouth, and has amazing powers of healing. The doctors and midwives will inspect your stitches to ensure that you are healing normally. Post-natal exercises will help to tighten the pelvic muscles around your vagina and although the soreness may last a little longer than after a normal delivery with no stitches, the vagina will heal and intercourse will soon be possible and satisfying (see Page 86).

In summary, therefore, with any difficult birth it is important to have an adequate explanation of the chain of events, and for the mother and father to participate in the birth where possible, and to be together with the baby as soon as possible afterwards.

Coping with a Sick Baby

If your Caesarean was performed because the baby was premature or was showing signs of distress, the baby may need to be nursed in a special care baby nursery or even transferred to an intensive care unit, which may not be in the same hospital. If you were awake at the time of delivery, the paediatrician will usually be able to let you see and hold the baby before taking it to the nursery, but if you are delivered under a general anaesthetic it will be a great shock to wake up and find no cot near your bed. This may increase the feeling of unreality that some women have about the birth, and this, coupled with anxiety about the baby's condition, may make the discomfort of the postoperative state seem almost intolerable.

Hospitals today realise the importance of keeping the mother informed, and will wheel you down to see the baby as soon as you can sit in a chair. Neonatal (which means newborn) intensive care units usually take a polaroid picture of the baby in its incubator, and send a paediatrician along to explain what all the tubes and wires attached to the baby are for.

Paediatricians now have the skill and the machines to help very sick babies recover, after a difficult delivery, from many of the conditions which used to kill them, and the long-term results are very good. However, this is a very anxious time for the parents, and sometimes confusion arises if different doctors try to explain complicated things using different words. Remember that you can always ask the consultant in charge to explain things if you are worried.

If the Baby Dies

About one Caesarean baby in a hundred will die, and although it is unusual after a planned Caesarean section to have a stillborn baby, a few may be malformed and die soon after birth. Women who have their babies early, or who develop severe high blood pressure or bleed heavily are much more likely to lose their babies than those who reach term, and as about four women out of five having Caesareans are at full term, they are more likely to have a live baby.

The death of a baby before birth may be even more difficult for the mother to accept than if the baby has lived for a few days. Psychologically, birth marks the change from the 'inside baby', a perfect idealised creature, part of the mother herself, and the real, crying, active baby—a person outside herself. If she does not see the stillborn child, especially if the birth has been by Caesarean or forceps under a general anaesthetic, it may be very hard to believe that she really has given birth and to start mourning the loss of the child.

Seeing and touching the dead child helps women to come to terms with their inner feelings and believe in the sad reality of the situation. Sadness, anger, disbelief, a feeling of guilt, physical symptoms such as a sinking feeling in the pit of the stomach, palpitations or dizziness, sleeplessness, loss of appetite and swings of mood are normal reactions to the death of a loved person, and the baby *is* a loved person to the parents. Your partner also feels the same way, but you and your partner may move through the different moods and emotions at different rates, which can cause misunderstandings. Doctors and midwives also feel a sense of failure, and may find it hard to repeat the explanations that the woman needs, but cannot take in or understand. The man usually has to register the death and make arrangements for the funeral, and generally cope with a stiff upper lip, and may feel that somehow it is his fault that the woman he loves has been damaged in the process of giving birth.

Most couples find the ritual of a funeral and burial or cremation helpful in marking the importance of the baby to them, and this can usually be arranged ten days or so after the delivery, so that the mother can attend. If she is not fit, most hospitals have a chaplain who will bless the stillborn baby or arrange some kind of service in the hospital for those that wish it.

Doctors will usually ask for a post-mortem to find out as much as possible about the baby's death, and most parents find this helps them in the task of trying to make sense of the death. A photograph of the baby, or mementoes such as the name band or a lock or hair, are kept and treasured by many couples, and you can ask the hospital to take a photograph if this is not offered to you.

It is only recently that doctors have really understood how seriously the couple may be affected by the death of a baby around the time of birth, but there is now more help available to help couples to come to terms with this sad experience. The Health Education Council produce a very helpful leaflet called *The Loss of Your Baby* (see Page 102).

6 Going Home

Seven to ten days after your Caesarean, you will be going home. Leaving hospital is an exciting moment, but beware—even a short journey can be exhausting. You will need to plan your life around your limited mobility for a while. If you have stairs, then make arrangements for everything you need to be on one level, so that you only have to make one journey up and down stairs each day. You are recovering from an operation as well as having to cope with the normal stresses and strains of having a baby, and you can expect to find life very tiring for a while. You will need all the help you can get!

Sleep

You will get tired easily. It can take anything from three to six months to recover all your old energy, simply because you have had a major operation. Do not set yourself high standards; take things slowly, and rest when the baby is asleep—do not use this as an opportunity to dash around cleaning. Tiredness can blow minor problems out of proportion. If you are breast-feeding, have the baby's cot next to your bed so that you can reach over without actually getting up. You may prefer to sleep with the baby in bed with you. There is no risk of suffocating the baby as nature seems to provide parents with an awareness while they are asleep, so the baby is safe. If you are bottle-feeding then enlist your partner's help for some of the feeds. He can also be very helpful if you are breast-feeding, picking up the baby and changing him or her ready for feeding, so that you can stay tucked up in bed!

Bleeding from the Vagina and Restarting Periods

By the time you get home you should not have any further fresh bleeding, but you may well have a pinky-brown discharge, which could last up to six weeks. Do not use any internal protection for the first six weeks because of the risk of introducing infection. Your first period will usually come one or two months after the baby's birth but if you are breast-feeding then you may not have a period at all, or you may just have a few spots of blood. By the time you have your first period it will be safe to use tampons again, if this is what you prefer.

Food

If you had a planned Caesarean you may have been able to stock up your cupboards or freezer beforehand. Rely on convenience foods for a while, and remember that if you are breast-feeding you will need plenty of fluids.

Washing Yourself

Always have someone around when you bathe at home for several weeks. You may find it physically difficult to get in and out of a bath alone; a stool or upturned bucket to sit on in the bath can be helpful. If you have a shower, this may be easier to use.

Washing Clothes

Your partner or friends could do the washing—and don't aim for perfection! You may only be able to keep up with the nappies some days. Delegate the ironing too, or else sit down if you do any yourself.

Changing the Baby

Find a flat surface at a suitable height for changing the baby so that you do not need to stoop. Disposable nappies can be helpful, especially in winter when it is difficult to dry towelling nappies.

Going Home

Shopping

Again, get help, and avoid carrying heavy baskets or bags for at least four to six weeks.

Housework

Don't aim for perfection—a bit of dust never hurt anyone. You will need help with the vacuum cleaner, changing beds, washing clothes, and so on. If you find problems in getting help, see if your doctor or social services department can arrange a home help.

Visitors

Make sure they let *you* sit down and hold the baby while *they* make the tea! Restrict your visitors to the few that you know will help, and with whom you can be honest and open. Too many casual visitors who need entertaining can be very tiring.

Toddlers

'Don't lift anything heavy' is easier said than done if you have another child who wants to share in your affections, and who may be feeling jealous of the new arrival. Dads and friends can be very helpful looking after the older children. Lifting a toddler after the first three weeks is unlikely to be dangerous, and kissing and cuddling are of course quite safe. Try to involve the older child in caring for the new baby and give a special cuddle at or after baby's feeding times.

Long separation from any child can lead to behaviour problems. The child may ignore you or be spiteful to the new baby; or it may regress to clinging and demanding behaviour. It is important to include the other child and also to find times when the new baby is asleep to give your attention completely to your other child or children.

Going back to work

If you have a job, you may not feel well enough to go back at the end of normal maternity leave. Consult your doctor before going back—he may recommend postponing your return.

Sex

Once the wound is healed and no longer tender, and the vaginal bleeding has stopped, you can make love and enjoy sex again. Sometimes tiredness and bad feelings about the birth can make it difficult for you to relax. About 10-20% of couples resume an active sex life before the post-natal visit at six weeks. After a difficult birth it is likely to take longer, but most couples are sexually active again three months after the birth. The frequency of intercourse may be less than before the pregnancy, because of tiredness, but most couples return to their pre-pregnancy enjoyment of sex in six months to a year.

There can be problems with sex after the birth; these can be related to pain from stitches in the vagina or fear of another pregnancy, or they can be more subtle subconscious problems because the woman has changed her role to become a mother. It can be difficult for either the man or the woman to come to terms with a sexual mother. If there are problems, talk about them with your partner and then with an understanding doctor, midwife or health visitor.

Local pain or discomfort in scar tissue can often be helped by using K-Y jelly to soften and lubricate the vaginal opening before intercourse. Pain during penetration can lead to a fear of love-making and put further stress on your relationship with your partner at this very vulnerable time.

Going Home

Contraception

A doctor will advise you before you leave hospital and your GP or family planning clinic can help counsel you afterwards.

The Pill. There are two sorts of pill. The combined oestrogen and progestogen pill is best avoided for the first six weeks because of your recent surgery and the risk of blood clots. It may also suppress breast milk. The progestogen-only pill can be taken first, and is safe for breast-feeding mothers. You can change onto the combined pill later.

The Coil. This can be fitted at your post-natal visit at six weeks.

Barrier Methods. Sheaths and pessaries are ideal to begin with. If you used a cap before delivery you will need to have the size checked as you may now need a bigger one.

Sterilization. Sometimes women request sterilization at the time of a Caesarean. Don't forget that the baby's survival to adulthood can never be guaranteed. Sterilization at the time of Caesarean carries a higher failure rate, so it is worth waiting several months before making such a big decision. Perhaps your partner might consider vasectomy?

Female sterilization can be done in two ways. The most common is using a small telescope-like instrument called a laparoscope. The laparoscope is put into the abdomen through a small hole made just below the umbilicus. The tubes can then be seen and then burnt or blocked with a small ring or clip. The other method involves making a small cut in the abdomen just above the pubic hair line and then cutting out a segment from each tube (tubal ligation). Both operations are done under a general anaesthetic. The stay in hospital is likely to be 48 hours after laparoscopic sterilization but could be 4-5 days after tubal ligation. If you are still breast-feeding, it is usually possible to bring the baby into hospital with you.

Post-natal Exercises

The physiotherapist will help and advise you in hospital; at home, following the advice in the booklet *You after Childbirth* (see reading list) will help.

Follow-up

Once you are at home, the midwife will visit you up to the tenth day, and can continue to visit up to the end of the first month. Your GP may also visit you, and after ten days the health visitor will call. She is a nurse especially trained to advise you about the baby's feeding, development, vaccinations, etc. She will follow your child's progress until he or she goes to school. You may also welcome the advice of a social worker if you have financial problems or are a single parent. Social workers can also help to arrange a home help if necessary.

Post-natal Check

If you had a difficult birth, you will probably have your six-week check-up back at the hospital. Write down all your questions before you go, as this is another good opportunity to find out 'why me?', and what methods of delivery to expect in your next pregnancy. You may have an X-ray of your pelvis taken so that its size and shape can be seen by the doctor and the possibility of a vaginal delivery considered for next time. If you are very small, then a repeat Caesarean will be necessary and this can be planned in advance.

Going Home

Future Pregnancies

After a Caesarean birth you would be wise to wait at least a year before becoming pregnant again, so as not to stretch the scar tissue too soon.

Future Deliveries

If you have a small pelvis you will need to have all your babies delivered by Caesarean: how many can you have? Most doctors would recommend that you stop at three, providing the babies are all healthy. If you are very keen you can have more babies, although there is a greater risk of the scar tissue giving way in late pregnancy, and the operation itself can become technically more difficult after many Caesareans. Some doctors will sterilize you at the same time as a third Caesarean but others would prefer to wait for six weeks to three months (see Page 87).

If your pelvis is a good size and shape, you will be able to go into labour next time and may well have a normal delivery. The labour will be watched carefully to make sure the progress is normal and thus the previous scar is not stressed unduly (see Page 40). Once you have had a Caesarean, a home birth would be most unwise.

7 Personal Experiences

Three very different Caesarean Births

When pregnant for the first time, nine years ago, the one thing I didn't want at all costs was a Caesarean section, having seen patients of my medical student husband looking ill and in pain while other new mothers bustled about the ward chatting. However, as the time drew nearer I thought no more about it and was dismayed when, after my waters had broken two days previously, the cervix had not opened and I was told I would need a Caesarean. The surgeon warned me that it would be painful and uncomfortable but that the one thing that would make it worthwhile would be the baby in the cot beside me.

That made sense, and anyway I thought it would be a relief to have the baby. However, I had never had an operation before and found the mask unbearable and the whole paraphernalia disturbing. Instead of a husband beside me, participating in the amazing experience of the birth of our first baby, I was alone among alien cloaked and masked figures.

The next thing I was aware of was a voice saying that I was to be thrown away and I felt myself to be small and, to all intents and purposes, dead, lying at the bottom of a dustbin. I looked up towards the light in time to see my husband putting the lid on the bin, but I could not make him see or hear that I was still alive. Leering faces came and went; the horror of those hallucinations experienced on regaining consciousness remained with me up to the birth of my second child, causing a certain amount of dread of further anaesthesia.

Someone told me I had a boy but I didn't see my baby for three days so I had none of the satisfaction of him lying beside me as promised by the surgeon. The pain was intense and my inability to move, apart from the excruciating effort of hoisting myself up by the bars of the bed head, was distressing, as was the constant need to lie on my back. The nights were especially bad; from being healthy, happy and excited after an uneventful and joyful pregnancy, I felt I had been reduced to a feeble invalid.

The baby, when he was eventually brought to me, seemed something alien and detached; he seemed not to be mine because I had not experienced his birth. In spite of the late start, I did feed Sam myself, although resting the baby on a tender stomach was sometimes excruciating. Recovery seemed much slower than that of my neighbours and even now when I hear others talk of the wonder of birth, I feel a sense of loss, an incompleteness that I was incapable of having a baby normally and could share none of the experiences of labour and birth with those around me.

My stomach was tender for some time and the operation left me prone to cystitis. I think, too, that a Caesarean is extra worry for the father, who can have no share in the birth. It also limits, to a certain extent, the number of births a mother can expect.

My second experience of a Caesarean beat the planned 'Elective Caesarean' by one day. Because of my worry that hallucinations might recur, I was offered an epidural instead of general anaesthetic. This I accepted only to retract after fellow patients persuaded me that it would be awful to be awake during an operation and to see what was happening, all of which I believed, stupidly, having never met anyone who had had a Caesarean by epidural. I was given a drug to bring me quickly back to consciousness so I avoided the hallucinations, only to suffer an ileus (failure of the bowel to work properly) on the third day after the operation. I also learnt that there had been problems during the anaesthetic and the doctors had had to operate very quickly to save Jessica.

I remember the horror of waking the first morning to find a dressing revealing a vertical wound that I felt would never allow me to wear a bikini again. Not only was it a long, vertical scar, but because Jessica had to be got out quickly and because of the ileus that followed, it was puckered, red and swollen. It

Coping with Caesarean

was embarrassing and ugly whereas the previous one had been low and horizontal with just a small drainage dent. Even now, I hate to see my stomach in the mirror, crisscrossed with lines.

When I was taken to see my baby the day after the birth, I could not imagine that she was mine—flabby, tube fed and dopey from the anaesthetic. The next few days I spent flat on my back after the ileus with tubes protruding from every orifice, only able to suck an ice cube and again with no baby in sight. After four days of this, I insisted on having my baby so that I could try, despite the tubes, to feed her. Gradually our relationship developed after its precarious start and I feel that, had she been my first baby, I would not have had the confidence to insist on her presence with me, and thus would never have successfully fed her or established any early contact with her.

After a second Caesarean I was even more protective of my scars, with an energetic two-year-old clambering over me at every opportunity. Everything physical suffered for some time, whether it was sexual relations, exercise or the day-to-day running of a home and family. With determination I managed and I don't remember ever being really depressed, but it was hard going.

In a vague attempt to exorcise the bad experience of earlier births, I longed for another child, determined this time to be in control, and to have as near natural a birth as I could. With the confidence of two previous Caesareans behind me and a greater knowledge of hospitals, I asked for a Caesarean by epidural. My husband was able to be with me so at last we could share the birth of our miracle baby. It was strange lying on the table knowing I was being cut open, yet feeling only a pulling and pushing, no pain. I asked my husband when the operation would start, only to be told that he could already see the baby's head! The birth itself took only minutes although the anaesthetic took a long time to administer but was far less frightening than a general, as I felt I could remain in control of what was happening and could at last participate in the birth. The moments I treasure are the ones of actually hearing my baby's first cry, hearing the words "it's a girl!" and holding her against my skin, covered as she was in blood and liquor, instead of being presented with a baby that was cleaned, polished and de-personalised in an incubator or cot as on previous occasions.

My feelings about her were incredible and still are, three years later, having seen her the moment she saw the world and having shared her birth with a loving and much-loved husband. She was always with me from then on. Neither of us had suffered the debilitating effects of the anaesthetic, so we enjoyed each other from the beginning. The pain, however, was even more excruciating once the epidural had worn off, perhaps because I had been sterilized at the same time. Nights especially were traumatic as I lay wondering if I dared to call a nurse yet again, or even if I could hoist myself up enough to reach the bell. In time the pain lessened, although I still suffered problems at home, with an infection in the tubes making housework and care of three children very difficult. Having Emily with me made up for everything—as my first surgeon had promised six years before!

This third birth also meant that my much resented scar could be excised and tidied up so that I feel happier in my bikini! A year after this birth I did have the scar injected by a plastic surgeon as it was still very pink and itchy. Now it is almost presentable and my only surviving problem is in telling my three beautiful children about the process of birth. "This is how a baby is born, BUT you came out a different way"!

Two Caesarean Births

When I was told that my first baby would need to be delivered by Caesarean (because of placenta praevia), my main feelings were of excitement and relief. Excitement because the nine long months of waiting and the *very* long last few days in the antenatal ward would be ended, no matter how abruptly. Relief because, ever since the moment when my GP had shaken his head over the baby's transverse position and decided to send me into hospital for checks, my husband and I had been suffering acute anxiety, the thought of malformation or still-birth very present in our minds (we had already had one late miscarriage). At last now something would actually happen and we would know the worst, or best. In fact the method of delivery seemed completely unimportant, compared to our worry as to whether the baby would be all right.

I was not unduly anxious about the operation itself, probably no more anxious than any first-time mother about the unknown experience of labour. However, it was irritating to be told by other expectant mums that I would be having a baby the easy way: just going to sleep and waking up to find the baby born, without any effort. I knew that there would be pain afterwards, even if I missed out on labour pains!

It is indescribably strange to go to sleep as one person and be woken an instant later (as it seems) as two people. Completely befuddled by anaesthetic, I was just able to understand that we had a daughter. She had breathing problems and was rushed to the Special Care Baby Unit. My husband saw her for a moment, but I don't remember doing so. Twenty-four hours later I was taken to the SCBU and, again, it was rather like a strange dream, to be taken into a room full of babies, and to look at them all, wondering which one was mine. I think I felt like an adoptive mother, being introduced to her future child. It was hard to believe she had been born from my body. However, we were lucky in that my husband and I could visit the SCBU any time, hold our baby's hand, touch her, cuddle her for a short time, and I was helped to breast-feed her. These early contacts were vital to dispel that first feeling of unreality and detachment, to bring home the fact that this was truly our baby.

Personal Experiences

For my son's birth I requested an epidural anaesthetic.
Beforehand there were the same feelings of excitement, but a
great deal more apprehension (I am very squeamish). My NCT
relaxation exercises helped greatly, and I felt I was playing
some sort of participatory role. Amazingly quickly, perhaps
after ten minutes, the surgeon announced "it's a boy!" and
handed me the baby. My feelings of joy and fulfilment were
more intense than any I have ever experienced before or
since; for two or three days I was on a wonderful "high", quite
drunk with delight in this new baby. I tried to put him to the
breast while on the operating table, pretty awkward while lying
flat and hitched up to drips, but we managed something. This
time there was no Special Care, no muzziness or sickness from
the anaesthetic. As soon as I was sewn up, we were simply
taken to the post-natal ward, as if it had been a normal
delivery, feeling happy and astonishingly well.

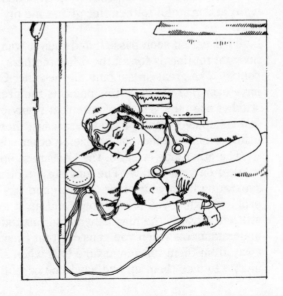

*It is perfectly
possible to feed
and cuddle the
baby while the
operation is still
going on and
you are being
stitched up*

Coping with Caesarean

The one person who really missed out was my husband, who very much wanted to be present at the birth of his children. Missing this experience has been a great sadness for him, although I don't think it has affected his very loving relationship with both of them. I must add that the hospital does allow fathers to be present at Caesarean births, although very few avail themselves of the privilege. I think, if our positions had been reversed, I would not have been able to watch him being cut up either.

I found no problems in breast-feeding my babies, given some pillows and some help lifting them to the breast at first. It is very frustrating though, to be unable to pick up your baby when you wish, without having to ring for a nurse. For the first couple of days after the operation I certainly felt convinced that I would split open if I made any sudden movements (I was terrified of sneezing!) and it was impossible to bend over to pick up the baby from its cot. The nurses were very busy, and I was dependent on the other mothers in the ward and grateful to them for giving me my baby when he cried.

That period soon passed, and then it was just the same hospital routine as for all the other mothers, but for longer of course. The great ordeal (and all the other Caesarean patients I have ever met agree on this point) is the dreadful day when the stitches are removed. I am sure that if any of the surgeons who sew us up ever had to have Caesareans, they might consider using soluble stitches, or find some other solution.

The other side effect of the Caesarean operation is the toll it takes on your family. The long stay in hospital involves long separation from your other children and this I think causes problems when you return home and must influence their attitude towards the new baby. Their attitude is very understandable when you consider that their mother is not only away from them for a long time but, when she returns, is unable to pick them up and has to be careful about many activities for the first three months at home. But these are minor problems. My two Caesarean operations have given me two beautiful, healthy children and really nothing else matters.

A Breech Birth

The birth of my second baby could easily have been by Caesarean as she was a breech delivery. It was a bit of a shock to be told the baby was in a breech position. I'd had a normal, straightforward pregnancy until 37 weeks when I thought the whole of my insides were rotating as my baby turned into this abnormal position. Whatever the reason, there was little space for her to turn back and there she remained until her birth three weeks later. It was strange to feel this obvious little head bobbing about where the kicking should be—I almost felt I could communicate verbally with this little creature.

My own doctor diagnosed a breech position, confirmed by a senior partner who also attempted to turn her externally. It was very uncomfortable as she was reluctant to be moved, so he decided to leave well alone and I was sent to see the Consultant. Fortunately he is a great believer in vaginal breech delivery wherever possible and an X-ray confirmed that my pelvis was big enough.

I needed to be mentally prepared to approach the birth with confidence, and I consulted as many people as possible about likely difficulties of a breech delivery. Entering hospital at 40 weeks I was well informed, and aware of the possible complications.

My labour was started off with a pessary to soften the cervix and by mid-morning I was on my way. I had asked for an anaesthetist to be present, to keep my options open for an epidural, which many of the medical staff had advised for a breech delivery. I was very dubious about this sort of anaesthetic, knowing it would immobilise me and had associated risks, but I was prepared to accept it if labour was hard, and for the sake of the baby's safe arrival, as a slow, careful delivery of the head is essential when the head is delivered after the body. I was also informed that forceps would almost certainly be used.

Labour progressed very rapidly with irregular, close contractions, and I had an extremely strong urge to push at only 3-4cm dilation of the cervix. I was aware that this could be a problem, as the baby's bottom is smaller than the head and is pushed into the opening cervix. I decided to have an epidural to help stop me pushing and to relieve the pain in my back. I was grateful for the relief the epidural offered but I was surprised to find I still had an overwhelming urge to push. I had a four-hour labour with periods of shakiness, sweatiness and fatigue and I wished it was all over and everyone would go away so that I could sleep.

As the second stage of labour began I was aware that this birth was anything but normal as it was to be witnessed by six student midwives, an anaesthetist and an obstetrician were on standby in case of an emergency Caesarean and a paediatrician was there to examine the baby immediately. The epidural was topped up as forceps were going to be used, but I was still able to feel my baby travel through the birth canal. I was hoisted in stirrups and baby's bottom appeared followed without difficulty by the legs and body; to help her I had been given a rather large episiotomy. It was a very tense moment for us as she was held by her legs and the forceps inserted and her head very carefully delivered, a perfect shape without damage.

Looking back, it was an exciting experience, although not as fulfilling as the birth of my first child, which was managed without drugs or epidural. The epidural worried me, especially as it took several hours for the numbness to wear off, due to the last-minute topping up. I was happy to have experienced the birth without the necessity of a Caesarean. My recovery was that of a normal birth with a little extra bruising from the forceps and episiotomy.

Personal Experiences

Some other quotes

On learning that a Caesarean Birth would be necessary:

"I was very upset because I wanted a normal birth. A Caesarean seemed too clinical, no mad dash in the middle of the night, no timing of contractions, is it—isn't it? However, once I had come to terms with the decision I made the best use of the days left and booked to have my hair done and had a night out with my husband the day before I had to go into hospital."

"I was totally unprepared and so the thought of going into an operating theatre filled me with horror. I was bitterly disappointed that I would not be able to deliver the baby myself."

"At 9.30 on Saturday morning I was told an emergency Caesarean would be necessary because the baby was distressed. I burst into tears—all those hours in labour."

During a Caesarean under epidural anaesthetic:

"In the end it was a marvellous experience: every care was taken setting up the epidural with explanations all the way, and I felt the anaesthetist was my true friend and ally. My husband was present and held my hands throughout. As Sarah was born I felt the sensations but not the pain and I saw Sarah immediately. There wasn't any sickness and I was conscious and alert all day until the evening sleep."

After a Caesarean Birth:

"I rather resented the baby and blamed him. I did feel cheated, as though I had been given a baby that could have been anyone's. I missed the actual first sight of the baby, knowing it was mine, the sense of relief and achievement and also my husband's company and pleasure. He found my having the operation a great strain, and not an experience he would like to repeat."

"There was quite a bit of pain to begin with but the hospital was very good and would give me painkillers when required."

"I couldn't move, it was too painful: I couldn't even reach the water. I called out but only a whisper came so no-one heard."

"Apart from an internal infection which I had for six weeks after the birth, I did get gradually back to normal, although for some weeks any clothing against the scar was very uncomfortable."

"I was very tired and felt poorly for a long time; the baby was unsettled for months. However, as time went on Andrew was much improved, and by 18 months I was much better and Andrew turned into a delightful boy."

"Baby Tom is 2½ years old and worth every minute of his difficult birth—more-or-less!"

Last Words

Between 1958 and 1970, the percentage of babies delivered by Caesarean almost doubled, from 2.7 to 4.5%, and from 1970 to 1978 the rate almost doubled again, to 8.7%. In some hospitals the proportion of women delivered by forceps may be as low as one in fifty, whereas in others it is as high as one in five. As nutrition has improved over the last 25 years and younger people are taller than their parents, one might have expected the rate of difficult delivery to fall rather than rise, but babies also tend to be bigger.

Nobody wants to return to the days when women laboured for days and an exhausted mother gave birth to a dead or handicapped baby, but as Caesareans have become safer, some doctors feel they are sometimes used too freely. If labour is induced before the woman is ready to deliver, it may fail and so a Caesarean is done; thus, very critical review of the indications for induction and the chance of it being successful will, it is hoped, reduce the number of Caesarean sections performed today. Monitoring the baby's heartbeat and testing the acidity of the baby's blood (see Page 24) together form a reliable method of detecting a baby in distress during labour, whereas monitoring the baby's heartbeat alone can be misleading and has been shown to increase the Caesarean section rate, without necessarily saving more babies. Some of the rise is explained by the ability of paediatricians to save very small babies; in the past most of these babies were unlikely to survive and therefore operating on the mother was not considered justifiable.

Pregnant women want to trust their obstetricians, and not to fight the medical profession, but doctors can hold very different views about the way to manage labour and delivery, and it is worth talking to your own GP about the policies of your local consultants. If you can't stand the idea of a long labour, and would like an epidural for pain relief, and to have your baby's heartbeat monitored continuously, then Consultant A may be the right person for you. If you want to start labour naturally, have no drugs and deliver in the squatting position, preferably without an episiotomy, then Consultant B may share your views.

Fortunately, in this country doctors do not perform operations because of the fees they will receive, and obstetricians are trained to do their best to assist women to have a healthy baby; so, once in labour, trust your doctor's judgement—he will be doing what is believed to be the best for both of you.

Useful Addresses and Further Reading

Useful Addresses

La Leche League of Great Britain, B.M. 3424, London WC1 6XX. Tel: 01-404 5011.
National Childbirth Trust, 9 Queensborough Terrace, London W2 3TB. Tel: 01-229 9319/9310.
Caesarean Support Group of Cambridge. Ann Watson, 7 Green Street, Willingham, Cambridgeshire.
AIMS (The Association for Improvements in Maternity Services). Elizabeth Cockerell, 21 Franklin Road, Hitchin, Hertfordshire SG4 0NE. Tel: 0462 2179.
Maternity Alliance, 309 Kentish Town Road, London NW5. Tel: 01-267 7477.

The Twins Clubs Association. Margaret Cann, Roma, Grange Road, Ash, Aldershot, Hampshire. Tel: 0252 310611.
Family Planning Information Service. Margaret Pyke House, 27/35 Mortimer Street, London W1A 4QW. Tel: 01-580 9360.
Mind (National Association for Mental Health), 22 Harley Street, London W1N 2ED. Tel: 01-637 0741.
The National Stillbirth Study Group, 66 Harley Street, London W1N 1AE.
Health Education Council, 78 New Oxford Street, London WC1A 1AH.

Further Reading

The Caesarean Birth Experience	B. Donovan, Beacon Press, 1978
The Experience of Childbirth	S. Kitzinger, Penguin, 1982
The Good Birth Guide	S. Kitzinger, Fontana, 1979
Pregnancy Questions Answered	G. Chamberlain, Churchill Livingstone, 1982
A Child is Born	L. Nilsson, Faber & Faber, 1981
Talking with Mothers	D. Breen, Jill Norman, 1981
The Experience of Breastfeeding	S. Kitzinger, Penguin, 1979
Breast-feeding after a Caesarean Birth	La Leche League International, Information Sheet No. 80
Nourishing Your Unborn Child	P. S. Williams, Avon Books, 1974
Essential Exercises in the Child-Bearing Year	Elizabeth Noble, Houghton & Miflin, 1976
Depression after Childbirth	K. Dalton, OUP, 1980
Our Bodies, Our Selves	A. Phillips and J. Rakausen, Penguin, 1978
The Womanly Art of Breast-Feeding	La Leche League International, 1981
A Mother's guide to breast-feeding and mothering the premature or hospitalized sick infant	La Leche League International, Information Sheet No. 109
New Life Book of Exercises for Childbirth	A. & J. Balaskas, Sidgwick & Jackson, 1979
The First Relationship: Infant and Mother	D. Stern, 1977
The Good Health Guide for Women	C. Cooke and S. Dorkin, revised British Edition, J. Turner & W. Savage, Hamlyn, 1981
The Birth Control Book	H. Shapiro, Penguin, 1980.
The British Way of Birth	E. Rantzen and G. Bourne, Pan, 1982
You after childbirth	J. McKenna, M. Polden and M. Williams. A Churchill Livingstone Patient Handbook
Twins	C. Zentner, Macdonald, Edinburgh, 1984